161 SEXUAL MYTHS

Clearing up a web of confusion

10 9 8 7 6 5 4 3 2 1

ISBN-10: 0-9890871-1-5
ISBN-13: 978-0-9890871-1-7
ISBN-13: 978-0-9890871-2-4 (ebook)

Printed and bound in U.S.A.

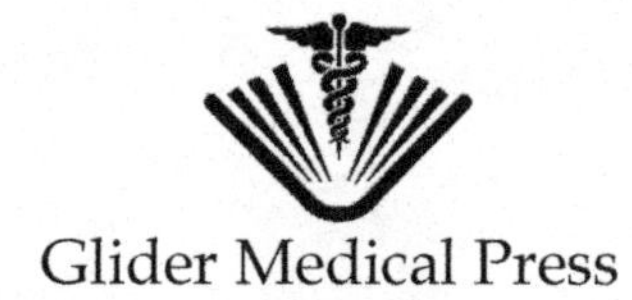

Glider Medical Press

161 SEXUAL MYTHS

Clearing up a web of confusion

JOSEPH I. EVANS, M. D.

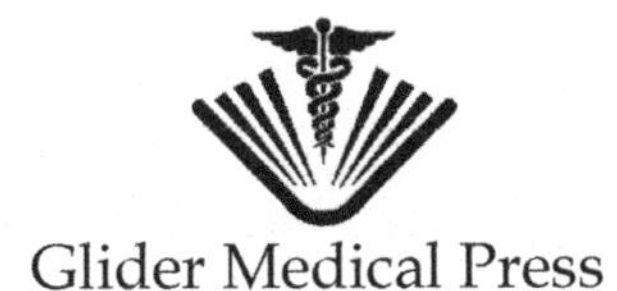

Glider Medical Press

ABOUT THE AUTHOR

Dr. Evans holds a B.Sc. degree from Clark College, B.Sc. Pharmacy from Florida A&M University School of Pharmacy, and Doctor of Medicine degree from the University of Miami.

His residency in Urology was done at Howard University, Washington, D.C. He did postgraduate studies in a number of prestigious academic institutions as well as specialized training in Tel Aviv, Israel.

Dr. Evans has over 40 years of professional experience and is a highly sought after health lecturer, having lectured in over 8 countries. He is a frequent guest on numerous radio and television shows.

For more information about Joseph I. Evans, M.D., visit www.drjosephevans.com

CONTENTS

INTRODUCTION

A myth is a commonly held incorrect belief. There are many sexual myths resulting in a web of confusion on sexual matters. Our thinking about sex is often influenced by our own personal biases, experiences, prejudices, religious beliefs, societal norms, local customs, and even gossip. The need for correct sexual information is especially acute among adolescents.

Some myths stated in this book may seem quite obviously incorrect to a reader. What is obvious to one person may be entirely inconspicuous to another person. There are individuals who take some myths very seriously, especially when they are stated by "responsible" persons. This is the reason why clearing up this web of confusion is so important. Misinformation and misdirected emotions can lead to unintended and dire consequences. This is especially true of sexual matters. Wrong facts can result in unwanted pregnancies, sexually transmitted diseases, and long lasting emotional scars. Some myths would seem comical, if the consequences were not so serious.

Making the correct decisions requires having the correct facts. This book is a compilation of commonly heard sexual myths. Some myths, as stated, are not grammatically correct but this is how they are usually spoken. The individual myth is listed then a factual rebuttal is given. The reader is given logical and scientific reasons for rejecting the myth. Extensive medical jargon is intentionally omitted. The information is intended to be understood by everyone and not just those with a medical background.

Despite the number of sexual myths presented here, believe me, there are more floating around out there. This listing of sexual myths is not exhaustive. However, a web of confusion will be cleared up by reading this book.

MALE AND FEMALE REPRODUCTIVE SYSTEMS

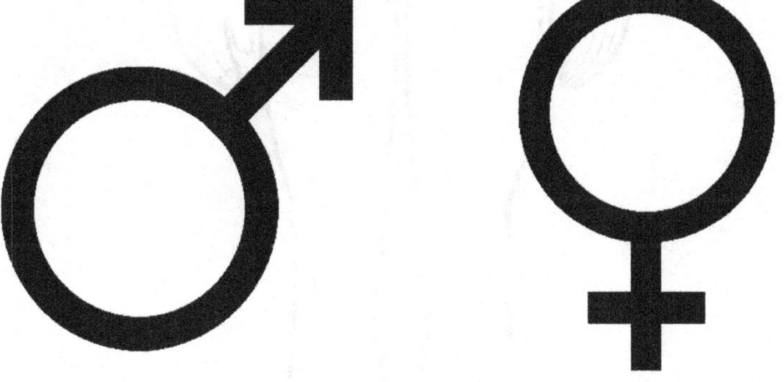

MALE ANATOMY

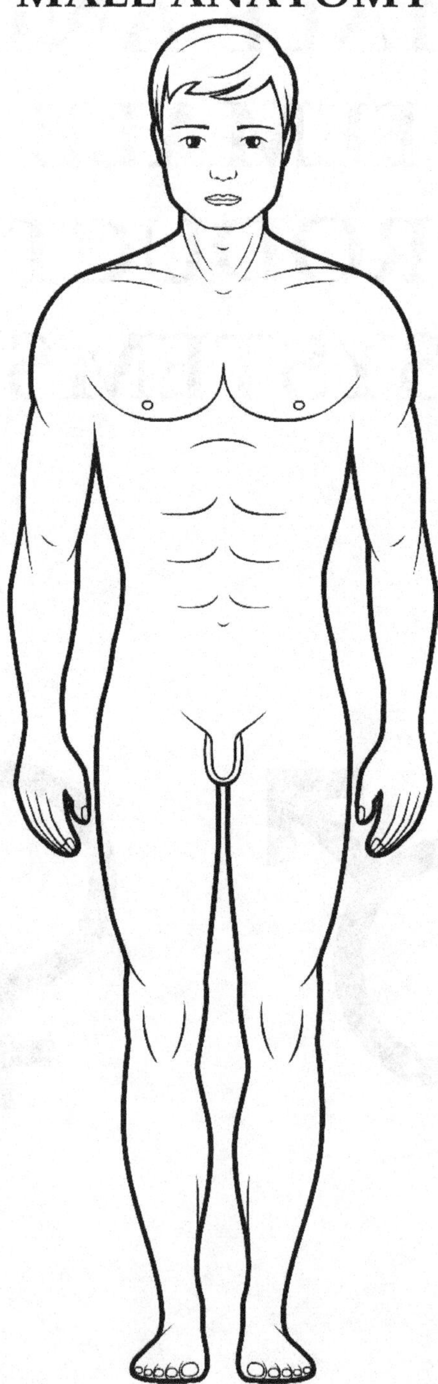

MALE REPRODUCTIVE SYSTEM

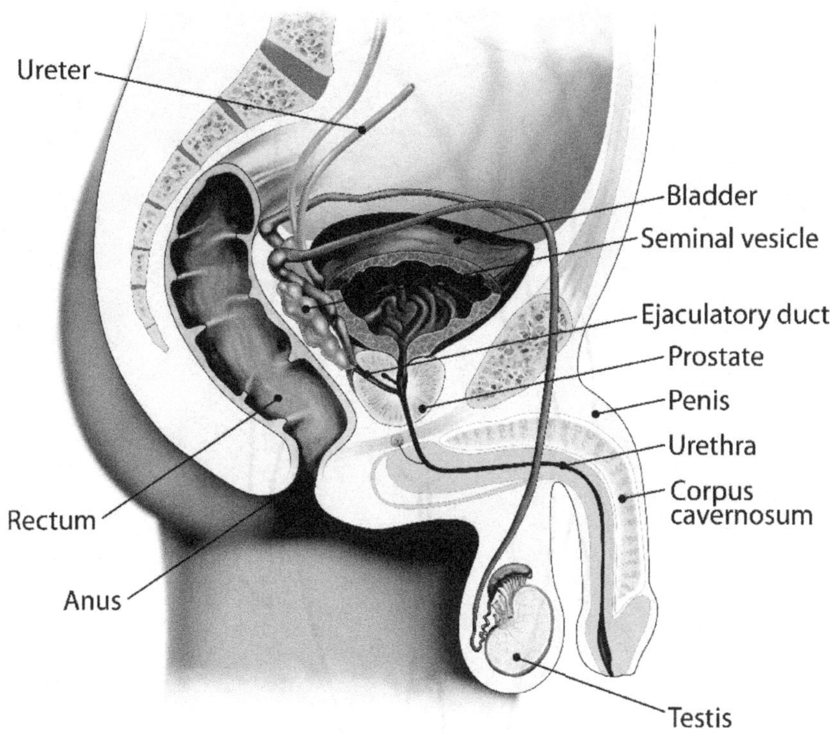

FEMALE ANATOMY

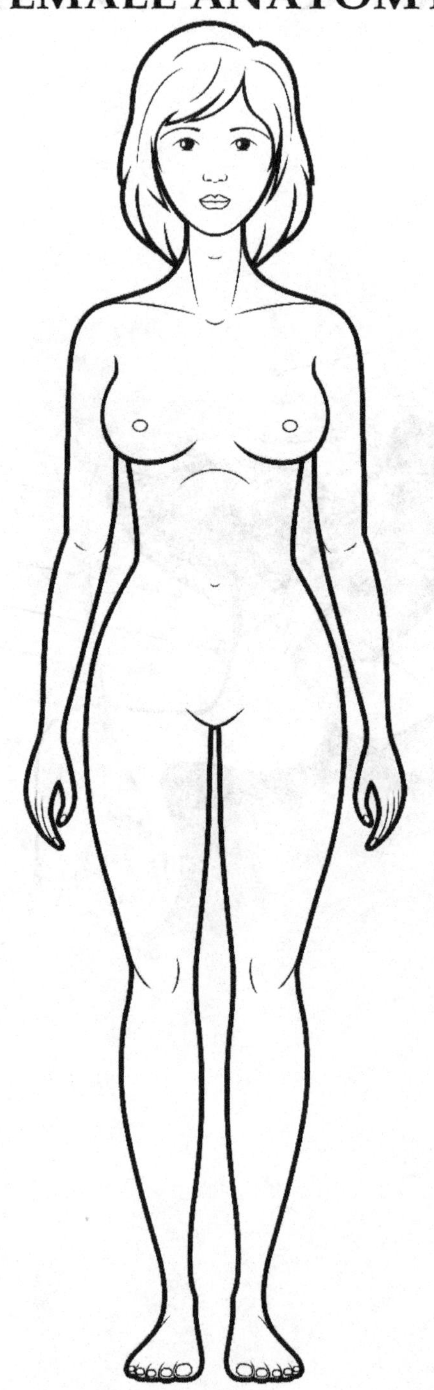

FEMALE REPRODUCTIVE SYSTEM

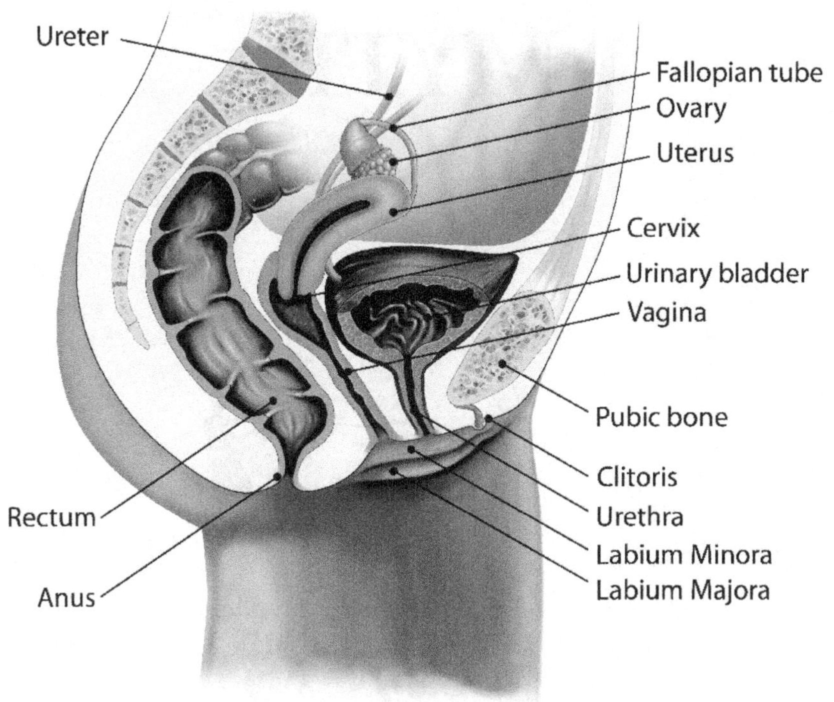

THE ANDROGYNOUS MYTH

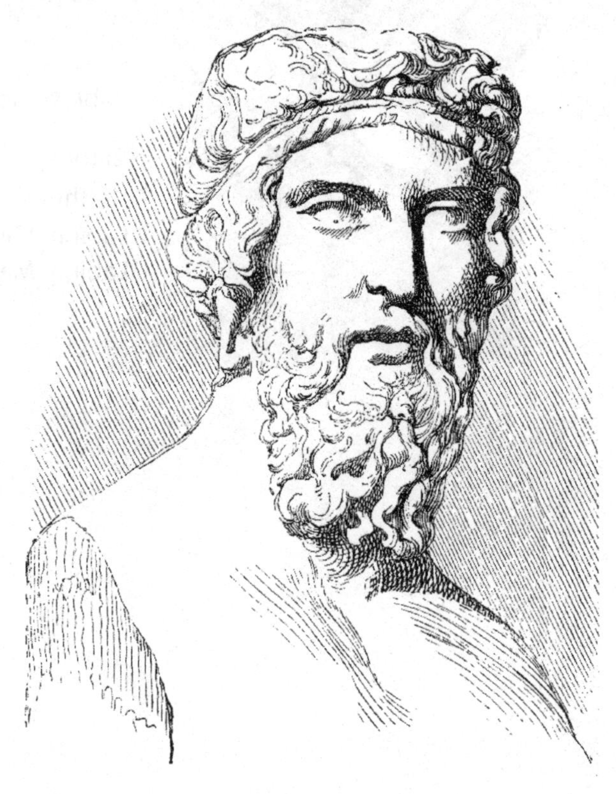

1

Males and females resulted from the dual nature of primal creatures. Some males attracted males and some females attracted females. Thus, love between like sexes is natural.

FACT:

Plato promulgated the above unnatural ideas, and even Aristotle, a student of Plato. The fact is that if you start with an erroneous premise, you are likely to end with an erroneous conclusion, as Plato did.

There is no evidence to show that male and female human beings ever existed in the same body or with dual natures. Even using the argument that there is an "undifferentiated stage" in fetal development would not suffice.

During early fetal development, there is a stage when physical characteristics of males and females appear similar. However, further analysis would show that the chromosomal makeup of the fetus is either male or female, unless there is a rare chromosomal anomaly. The distinction between male and female existed prior to conception, that is, in the sperm and egg.

As far as human knowledge permits, there is, and always has been, and no doubt always will be a distinction between male and female human beings. We can distinguish male and female by chromosome and DNA analysis today, and even simply by the "carrying angle" of the upper extremities. Aberrations do occur rarely, but only rarely.

Males and females obviously serve different functions, otherwise nature would have no need for both. This does not negate the fact that a person may feel attracted to anyone or anything. Persons with fetishes are not proof that the fetish was once a part of human nature.

Male and female are naturally complimentary. Nature has provided the means for this to happen physically, and emotionally.

MALES AND SEXUAL MYTHS

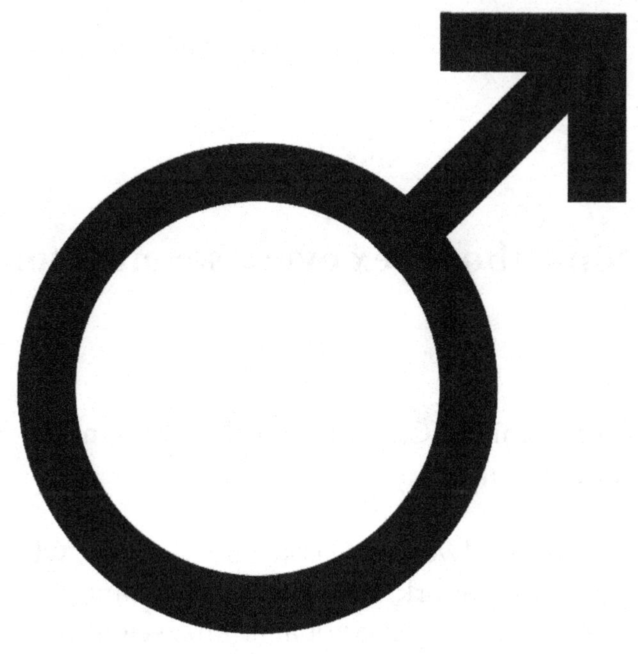

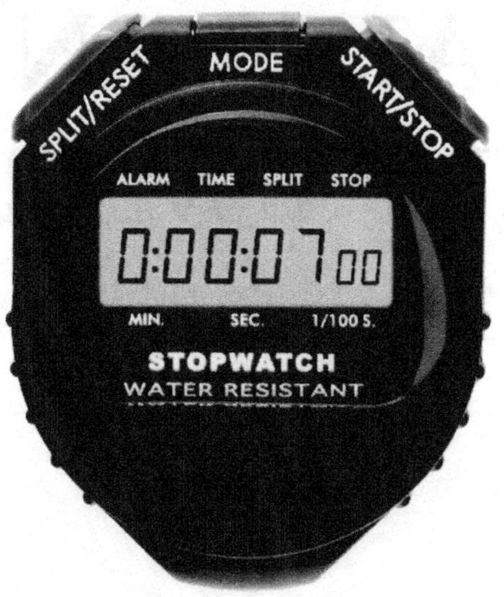

2

Men think about sex every seven seconds.

FACT:

What an active mind! Can this explain why some men don't get anything done?

If a man's mind is always and constantly on sex, when does he think about family, work, school, church affairs, recreation, civic affairs, politics, international affairs, scientific research, etc., etc., etc.

Imagine a surgeon performing a major operation, or a pilot flying a jumbo jet loaded with passengers, or an astronaut on his way into space. I know from personal experience that sex is farther away during such activities than the moon.

I don't know who did the measurements on how often men think of sex, but every seven seconds? This is highly suspect!

There are many professions that require paying strict attention to details, sometimes for extended periods of time. Deviation from the task at hand, even mentally, can result in a catastrophe. Consider the work of virtuoso violinists in a concert, musicians during a half-time show at a football game, scientists engaged in classified nuclear research, air traffic controllers at a busy international airport, or as in my case, doing surgery deep in the human body. These activities and other such tasks, do not allow for frivolous thinking every few seconds, or every few minutes either!

3

Men are always ready and always want sex.

FACT:

A man's desire for sex may be influenced by many factors, such as stress, medical status, medications, interpersonal relationships, religious taboos, work, school activities, attractiveness of his partner or lack thereof, etc.

Imagine a man watching a championship basketball game. The score is tied, ten seconds to go in the game. His favorite team has the ball. Do you think he is ready for sex at that moment? A scantily clad model would be likely to have no appeal at that point in time.

For many men, "the moment must be right."

4

Men want sex more than women do.

FACT:

Men do not have a monopoly on sex. Men and women are both sexual beings. The desire for sex is alive and well in women as much as it is in men.

Due to hormonal changes, some women may have varying levels of desire for sex at different times of their lives.

There are many factors affecting a person's libido, including the following:

- Stress
- Medication
- Health status
- Hormone balance or deficiencies
- Mental status
- Interpersonal relations
- Physical impairments
- Self-confidence, and lack of self- confidence
- Diet
- Sleep patterns

5

The male always initiates sexual advances.

FACT:

There may have been a time when this was true, but not in today's world.

In this age of liberated females and personal freedoms, women "have come a long way, baby." It is not unusual, now, for a woman to approach a man covertly or overtly.

In some places males are markedly outnumbered by females. A woman may find herself being very aggressive, thinking that she may be "left behind" if she waits to be approached by a man.

Even among dedicated couples it is not unusual for sexual advances to be initiated by the female.

6

A man is better off being single.

FACT:

There are advantages and disadvantages in everything, including being single.

The Journal of Epidemiology and Community Health reports that a 2008 study showed that married men are healthier and wealthier. It has been known that sexually active men tend to live longer.

Being single may mean fewer expenses, as compared to having a family, with a wife and children. This may be fine with some individuals. There are persons who would be unfulfilled in life being alone in adulthood.

Human beings are social beings. We generally need one another, for one reason or another. That is why God was quoted as saying, "It is not good for man to be alone." Marriage has proven itself to be the strongest bond for companionship. It has also been proven to be the basic and fundamental unit of society.

If a man wants to remain single, especially after a failed marriage, he may very well find peace in being single. However, as a general position in life, "God knows best."

7

Masturbation is a male activity.

FACT:

Masturbation is a human activity, being common among both males and females. It has become so common among females that there are now specialized accoutrements for them to accomplish the act. The sale of these items has become a virtual industry in itself.

8

Too much masturbation will shrink the penis.

FACT:

Penis size is determined by genetics and influenced by hormones.

The exercise of masturbation will not determine penis size, nor will it change the size of the penis.

9

Masturbation can make the penis bigger.

FACT:

Not so. If this exercise could enlarge the penis there would be more "giants" in the land. There is no relationship between masturbation and penis size.

Penis size is determined genetically and influenced by hormones, especially during infancy.

10

Masturbation causes blindness.

FACT:

If this were true, there would be more blind men and women around. There is no known direct connection between the penis, or vagina, and the eyes.

There is no scientific evidence linking masturbation and blindness, deafness, hairy palms, mental illness, or impotence. Nor will it cause curvature of the erect penis, as many people believe. Angulation of the erect penis may likely be due to Peyronie's disease, a problem wherein a scar tissue-like plaque forms in a subcutaneous layer in the penis.

11

No penis is too large for any vagina.

FACT:

The vagina is adaptable, such as during childbirth. The hormonal and tissue changes that take place during foreplay are different from those that take nine months to prepare the birth canal during pregnancy.

All vaginas are not the same size. A specially endowed penis can cause discomfort and trauma to a less endowed vagina. A snug episiotomy repair after childbirth can also limit the acceptance of King Kong. This is also a reason why child molestation is such a heinous crime.

12

The bigger the penis, the better the sex.

FACT:

This is a very popular myth, but bigger is not necessarily better. A well-endowed man, using poor technique, can cause discomfort rather than pleasure. Some men with large organs are inclined to engage in deep thrusting, often resulting in vaginal abrasions and cervical bruising.

Nerve endings in the vaginal area are concentrated in the lips and outer portions of the vagina. This can explain why women may enjoy less endowed males. After all, "it's not the size of the ship, it's the motion in the ocean." Occasionally though, there is the woman who prefers Mr. King Kong.

13

If a man doesn't cum during sex his testicles will burst or explode.

FACT:

This myth is especially popular among sexually inexperienced males. Most men have experienced sex without ejaculation at some point during their lives but their testicles did not burst or explode.

The excitation of sexual stimulation, increased pelvic blood flow, pelvic muscular contractions, seminal fluid production and sperm movement, all lead to resolution by ejaculation. In the absence of ejaculation, a feeling of fullness anywhere in the pelvic region, including the testicles, may occur. The testicles may even become painful. The impression that the testicle may burst is very misleading.

The testicles are contained in a very durable sheath called the tunica albuginea. The tunica is tough enough that rupturing during normal sexual intercourse is most unlikely. Rupturing is more likely to occur with direct trauma to the testicle.

14

Wet dreams occur only in males.

FACT:

Females also experience spontaneous nocturnal orgasms, or wet dreams. The trigger of these events has not been identified.

15

The head of the penis must be hard for a good erection.

FACT:

The penis is made up of three cylinders. Two of the cylinders are filled with spongy tissue. During erection, the spongy tissue fills with blood, becoming quite rigid.

The third cylinder contains the urethra through which urine flows. The end of this cylinder expands into what is known as the glans penis, or head of the penis. The glans penis also covers the ends of the two spongy cylinders.

During erections, the rigidity of the spongy cylinders can push against the head of the penis hard enough to make the glans penis feel hard also. These two spongy cylinders, called corpora cavernosa, are responsible for the hardness of the erection. The other cylinder, called the corpus spongiosum, is not primarily responsible for the rigidity of the erection.

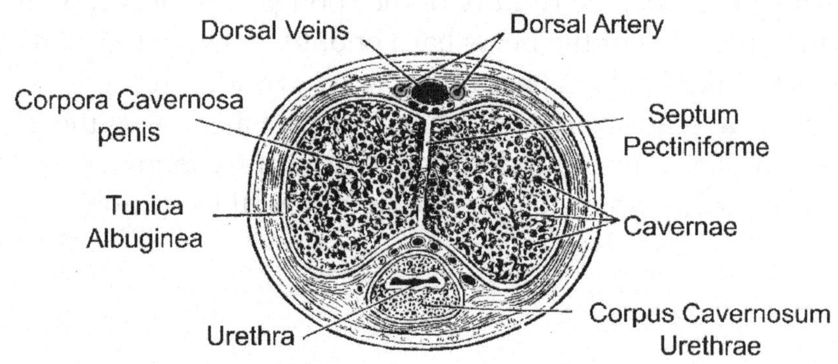

16

There's no such thing as a broken penis.

FACT:

Oh yes, there is!

The penis can be fractured. This usually happens during vigorous sexual activity, while the penis is erect. In a significant number of cases it happens with the female in the dominant position during sex.

When the penis is fractured, there may or may not be immediate pain. There is often a "popping" sound and loss of erection when this happens. Due to the "break" in the tough tissue surrounding the corpus cavernosum, called the tunica albuginea, bleeding may occur under the skin of the penis. This can cause swelling in the penis.

If a fracture occurs, or is suspected, the man should seek immediate urological attention for assessment and management of the fracture.

17

The penis gets bigger when you lose weight.

FACT:

Losing weight from the fat pad over the mons pubis (fat pad above the penis) allows the penis to be more obvious. The phallus, or body of the penis, doesn't actually grow or get bigger when body weight is lost. So, losing weight might be good for allowing the penis to be more apparent.

18

The penis gets significantly shorter after having a circumcision.

FACT:

The circumcision removes redundant foreskin from the penis. It does not shorten the phallus, or body of the penis. The length of the penis is the same before and after the circumcision. Perhaps, the "bare" appearance of the glans penis (head of the penis) gives the illusion of a shorter penis. A patient told me that his penis got five inches shorter after having his circumcision. He claimed to have had ten inches prior to the circumcision. Talk about a tall tale! This is the stuff that myths are made of. He was probably influenced by the common tale among men prior to circumcision that says, "It won't be long now!"

19

Height, nose, feet, hands, or fingers indicate the size of a man's penis.

FACT:

These structures do not determine a man's penis size. Just as these physical attributes are inherited, so is penile size. Looking at a fully clothed tall, short, thin, or fat man would not give a clue as to his penis size.

Hormonal influences during embryonic development, and postnatally, may also play a role in determining penis size. Also, the penis is not a muscle as some may claim. Thus, it does not hypertrophy from frequent and strenuous use.

20

Taking a sex pill gives a man an erection.

FACT:

An erection is a complex hemodynamic event. No pill can meet all of the requirements for producing an erection. Medication and supplements can assist a man with achieving an erection, especially by increasing blood flow to the penis. Most "sex pills" work by increasing blood flow to the pelvic region, including the penis. Another important component for achieving an erection is the desire for sex.

Required parameters for normal erections include:

1. Normal penile anatomy
2. Intact, functioning nervous system
3. Unimpeded vascular, or blood flow
4. Adequate endocrine functioning, i.e, hormones
5. Psychological well-being

It is interesting to note that the psychological parameter can actually override all of the others. Here's an example: John is watching a 15 round heavyweight championship fight. The fight is now at 30 seconds to go in the 15th round and thus far an even fight between the two fighters. Suddenly, John's favorite boxer lands a left uppercut to the chin and a right cross to the head of his opponent. The opponent stumbles. At that very moment John's scantily clad wife walks into the room.

No pill in the world could give John an erection at that moment! His psychological parameter would not allow the others to work at that moment. Incidentally, John had not noticed the bikini clad girls holding the ring sign between rounds either.

Medication, currently available, act primarily by increasing blood flow to the penis. In some situations, medication may be given to correct a specific medical abnormality.

21

A man's erection lasts longer if he wears a condom.

FACT:

This may very well occur in an individual case, but wearing a condom won't make a difference in most men. If a condom would prolong erections condoms would be recommended for premature ejaculations.

22

Testosterone is the only hormone that is important in a man's sexuality.

FACT:

Testosterone may be the dominant hormone in a man's body, sexually, but other hormones are important also. These other hormones include growth hormone, prolactin, estrogen, dehydroepiandrosterone and luteinizing hormone.   Each hormone has specific actions in the body. Even the ratio of one hormone to another can affect a man's sexuality.

23

If a man has only one testicle his children will be all boys.

FACT:

There is no scientific evidence that having only one testicle would produce only Y chromosome sperm or only X chromosome sperm. Thus, any testicle can be expected to produce X and Y chromosome sperm. I have never heard or read of a man who produces only X or Y chromosomes. The female egg contains only X chromosomes. The male sperm contains X and Y chromosomes. When the chromosome from the male sperm combines with the chromosome from the female egg, the resulting fetus will be of the sex depending on whether the sperm contributed the X or Y chromosome.

A fetus with XX chromosomes would be a female. A fetus with XY chromosomes would be a male.

There are situations where all offspring are males or females in a family. The presence of both testicles or the absence of a testicle is not the deciding factor in these families. Mathematical probability dictates that such inheritance will occur now and then. There may be an unknown genetic factor influencing the chromosome selection but it is certainly not the presence or absence of a testicle.

Just imagine, is this were true, a man with two or three daughters and desiring a son, would only have to remove a testicle and ----bingo----the rest of his children would be boys.

A patient told me that one of his testicles was surgically removed during his boyhood. The doctor told him that as an adult he would only be able to produce boys. He later fathered four boys and no girls. He felt, however, that he had all boys due to "chance alone."

Simple illustration of X and Y chromosome combinations from sperm and egg.

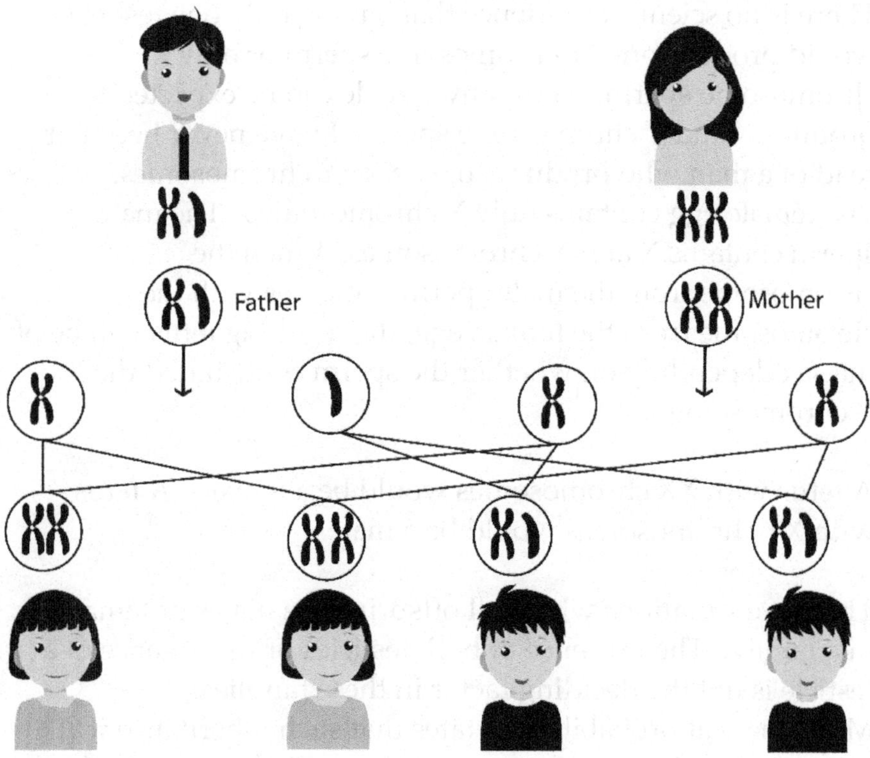

Note that in any pregnancy there is a 50% chance of having a male or female baby. All other factors involved in gender selection, other than chance, are unknown.

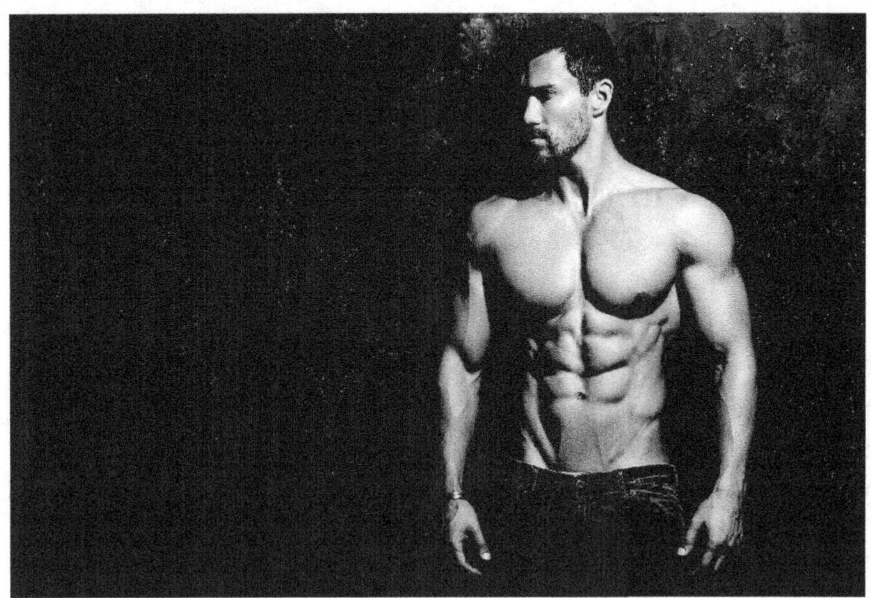

24

A virile man is very fertile.

FACT:

There is no relationship between virility and fertility.
A virile man may be very active, very macho and shoot many blanks! His testicles may be incapable of producing sperm or sufficient numbers of sperm. Male fertility refers to a man's ability to produce children. It is his ability to produce sperm that can fertilize the female egg. His fertility is dependent upon his hormone levels, health of the testicles, and the quality and quantity of the sperm produced.

Note that muscular development and physique, sexual performance and even intellectual acumen have nothing to do with a man's fertility status.

25

Men cheat more than women.

FACT:

Cheating may involve various types of relationships, such as physical, emotional or financial. This myth refers to physical infidelity in a heterosexual relationship where the man cheats with another woman or the woman cheats with another man.

Numerous surveys have been done to settle this issue. Some of the factors influencing survey outcomes include the following:

- Some research is skewed to men, others are skewed toward women
- Men tend to be older than female partners
- Men tend to be more financially independent
- Women are less likely to admit to cheating

According to the Journal of Marital and Family Therapy infidelity statistics are similar for men and women. A considerable fact is when a man cheats, a woman is involved, and conversely, a cheating woman does so with a man. Of course, in 21st century living, cheating involves same sex and heterosexual infidelity.

26

Most cases of impotence are due to psychological causes.

FACT:

Only about 10% of cases of impotence are due to psychological causes. Most cases have an organic basis. Some causes of impotence include diabetes mellitus, hypertension, anti-hypertensive medications, hormonal imbalances, prostatitis, prostate cancer, cardiovascular disorders, neurologic disorders, pelvic surgery or trauma, and various drugs.

There is also the issue of the andropause. This refers to the decline of hormone levels as men get older. The hormonal decline is gradual and is often not noticed by many men. There are physical changes in the male body that accompany the decrease in hormone levels.

One of the most recognized change in older men is a decrease in libido. This is due to a decrease in testosterone, often coupled with medical problems as well.

Note that the andropause occurs gradually over several years. The menopause in females occurs more precipitously and is more easily recognized.

27

An older man, for example, in his 80's, cannot produce a pregnancy.

FACT:

Many men are capable of producing sperm well into old age. Records of older men fathering children go back at least to biblical times. Modern records confirm the same.

Currently, in medical history, where hormone replacement therapy and anti-aging protocols are common, the reproductive life span of males is likely to be extended.

28

Large quantities of semen make a man more sexual.

FACT:

During ejaculation, a man is usually unaware of the volume of his ejaculate. Furthermore, ejaculation occurs toward the end of the physical action of intercourse. The remainder of love making is not dependent upon semen volume.

The amount of semen varies from person to person, and even from time to time in the same individual. Rather than semen volume, a man's sexuality is more dependent on his own physical prowess, experience, emotions, social trends, religion, and response to his sexual partner.

29

Large quantities of semen make a man more fertile.

FACT:

More is not always better!

Semen volume does not determine a man's fertility. Sperm quality is the determining factor. Important aspects of sperm quality include the sperm count, sperm morphology and sperm motility. Other factors which may also affect a man's fertility include things such as his medical and nutritional status, medication, and genetics.

The main function of the prostate gland is to produce the liquid portion of semen, called seminal fluid. This function is independent of sperm production. Sperm are produced in the testicles, transported to the area of the prostate via the little tubes called vas deferens, where they are mixed in the seminal fluid. This is ejaculated as semen.

The seminal fluid also provides nutrition for the sperm. A man may generate a large volume of semen that contain few sperm (oligospermia) or no sperm at all. (azoospermia). This may be due to a previous vasectomy, pelvic surgery, medication or drugs, an illness, low hormone levels (hypogonadism), testicular tissue abnormalities, or other unknown reasons.

Azoospermia is popularly known as "shooting blanks."

30

A man can judge his fertility by the volume and thickness of his semen.

FACT:

This is a common myth among men.

The volume and thickness of semen do not determine a man's fertility status.

His fertility status is more influenced by his hormone levels and quality of sperm. Hormones which influence male fertility include prolactin, testosterone, luteinizing and follicle stimulating hormones.

The sperm count, motility and morphologic features of the sperm influence sperm quality. The sperm count refers to the number of sperm per milliliter of semen. This is also known as sperm concentration.

I have seen men with large volumes of semen and only a few sperm (oligospermia) or even no sperm at all (azoospermia). This can occur, for example, in men who smoke marijuana. This can also occur in men whose testicles are deficient in the cells that produce sperm.

31

Only older men get erectile dysfunction.

FACT:

Erectile dysfunction can occur at any age. The incidence increases with advancing age but is likely to be related to cardiovascular compromise and hormonal changes. A decrease in hormone levels is also common in older men. By the age of 70 about 80% of men experience this problem. Therefore, many people think that erectile dysfunction is a problem of old age. However, I have seen men in their 20's and 30's with this problem.

Quite often erectile dysfunction is only a symptom of an otherwise undiscovered medical condition. The evaluation of erectile dysfunction may be a lifesaving process.

The following are some of the causes of erectile dysfunction:

- Diabetes
- Hypertension
- Cardiovascular disease
- Neurological disorders
- Medications
- Chemotherapy
- Untreated priapism
- Pelvic trauma, including pelvic surgery
- Prostate cancer
- Alcohol, marijuana, and cocaine use

- Psychological factors
    o Anxiety
    o Depression
    o Guilt
    o Stress

32

Only men experience sexual dysfunction.

FACT:

Sexual dysfunction in males may include loss of libido, impotence, premature loss of erections, premature ejaculation, and priapism.

Women have sexual dysfunctions as well, including loss of libido, anorgasmia, dyspareunia, and vaginismus.
Loss of libido refers to a lack of interest in sexual activity. This may be due to stress, depression, lack of rest, medication, problems in interpersonal relations, illness, decrease in hormonal levels, or any other reason. Loss of libido occurs in both men and women.

Impotence is the inability to achieve or maintain an erection satisfactory for sexual intercourse. There are many causes of impotence. Most cases of impotence have an organic basis rather than a psychological basis. Impotence may be a symptom of a serious underlying problem. This is the reason why a proper health care provider should evaluate impotence. Premature ejaculation is experienced by most men at some point in time. It can be frustrating to a man as well as to his sexual partner. Premature ejaculation may occur spontaneously but can be brought on by anxiety or depression, inflammation in tissues and infections.

Priapism is a persistent or prolonged undesired erection. This potentially painful condition is actually a medical emergency, requiring expert management.

Anorgasmia is the lack of orgasms. Many women do not experience an orgasm. Note, however, that an orgasm is not necessary to enjoy sexual activity, nor is it necessary for pregnancy to occur.

Dyspareunia refers to painful intercourse. This can be due to hormonal imbalances resulting in tissue dryness, thus requiring an appropriate lubricant or correction of the condition. This may also be due to various medical conditions or simply physical incompatibility.

Vaginismus is the persistent involuntary contraction of vaginal tissue or pelvic muscles in females. This can be annoying if it occurs at the wrong time.

33

Prostate surgery always results in impotence.

FACT:

The effect of prostate surgery on a man's potency depends upon the kind of surgery performed.

Prostate surgery for bladder obstruction is unlikely to cause impotence. Sex after surgical recovery should be as good as before surgery. Sometimes, there is retrograde ejaculation after this kind of surgery. In retrograde ejaculation, the semen falls back into the bladder and is expelled in the urine during urination. There is no interference with erections, ejaculation, or the sensations of ejaculation.

Prostate surgery for cancer of the prostate may or may not cause impotence. The effect on potency depends upon the surgical technique used, the extent of the cancer, as well as the skill of the surgeon. Sometimes it is impossible to remove all of the tissue that needs to be taken without damaging the nerves that control a man's potency.

Nerve sparing radical prostatectomy, popularized by Dr. Patrick Walsh of Johns Hopkins University, raised awareness among urologists of preserving a man's potency during prostate cancer surgery. Dr. Sanjay Razdan, of the International Robotic Prostatectomy Institute, Miami, Florida, is pioneering a technique of nerve preservation using amniotic membrane tissue during laparoscopic removal of the prostate. A recent finding is that starting on appropriate medication soon after surgery helps to maintain erectile function.

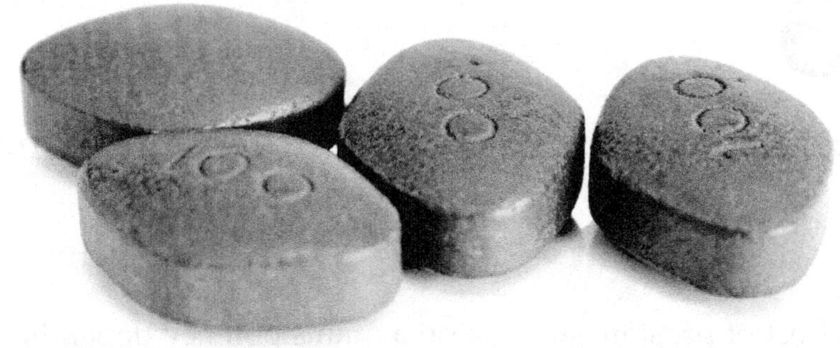

34

An older man would die if he takes Viagra and has sex.

FACT:

Viagra contains an active ingredient called sildenafil. One of the actions of sildenafil is to increase blood flow to the penis thereby facilitating a penile erection.

Since Viagra was introduced to the public in 1998, many older men have used it successfully and safely. I have prescribed sildenafil for many men, of all ages.   I have not had any reports of serious adverse effects from sildenafil use. There are now other compounds similar to sildenafil also being used safely.

Imagine a 75-year-old man, with heart failure, who has not had an erection or sex for the past 15 years. He takes Viagra and gets an erection. It can even relieve his chest discomfort. This eager beaver grabs a 25-year-old fire-fly. Not only does he try to keep up with her, but, he tries his best to give her a manly impression. He dies between Act 1 and Act 2!

Of course, the fire-fly would blame the death on Viagra. She would never admit that her robust sexual escapade was too much for the old man. His death was likely due to over exertion, regardless of whatever aided him in getting the erection. This fellow should have checked with his physician for proper evaluation and instructions before taking his terminal wild ride.

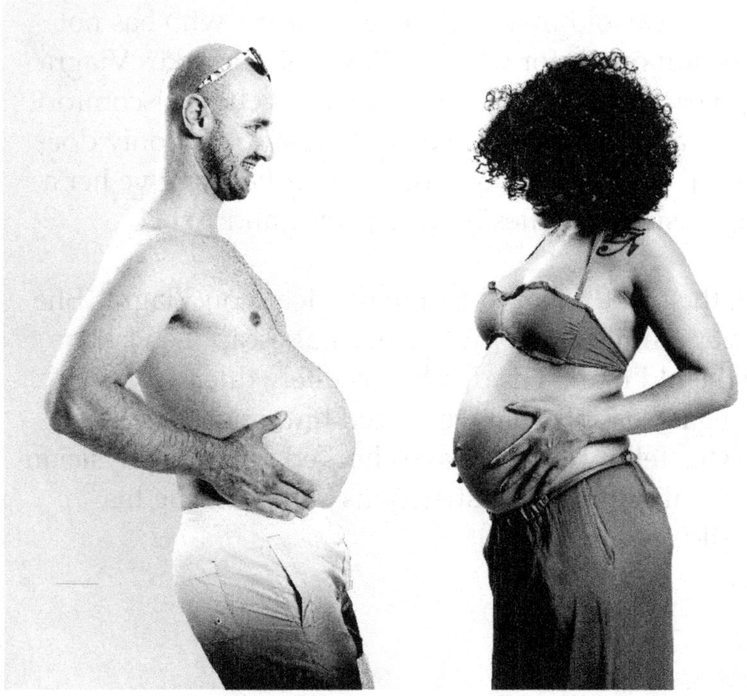

35

It is now possible for men to get pregnant and have children.

FACT:

No, No, No!

To date, it is not possible for men to get pregnant or bear children. There are scientists who are interested in bringing this about. It would take another book to list all of the reasons why men cannot get pregnant or bear children, but here are just a few:

- Wrong genetics. The male body is genetically engineered for male functions, which excludes pregnancy. The male reproductive system, as inherited at the moment of conception, excludes the anatomy and functions of a female reproductive tract.
- No ovaries, thus no egg
- No fallopian tubes, thus no fertilization of the egg
- No womb, thus no endometrium, that is, no implantation of a fertilized egg. No menstrual cycle without the endometrium, thus, no fertile days. No development of a placenta without the endometrium. The placenta attaches the unborn baby to its mother and supplies nutrients and everything else for the developing baby. In vitro fertilization with implantation into the hostile male abdomen won't work either.
- No birth canal. The stork may just have to bring the baby!
- Wrong physical, biochemical and hormonal environment
- Wrong emotional makeup. It is said that women remember the pain of childbirth but forget the suffering of childbirth. Many believe that men will never forget the pain or the suffering of childbirth. This indicates a possible difference in the psyche of males and females.
- The male pelvis is not architecturally or dynamically suitable for child bearing and delivery
- Male breasts are not designed for milk production
- Male pregnancy would eliminate the need for love making between males and females. This is a possible

explanation as to why Eve was made for Adam's companionship instead of another male.

- The male body is designed to complement the female body, not replace it.

36

Men can bleed after sex, so men have periods too.

FACT:

In females, the uterus, or womb, is uniquely designed to receive a fertilized ovum. This capability is renewed approximately each month in the non-pregnant female. The fertilized ovum is the combination of the male sperm and the female egg.

The lining of the uterus, or the endometrium, builds up between menses. This is necessary for providing the proper developmental environment for the fertilized ovum. There are numerous hormonal and biochemical changes that occur in the female body that produce these changes in the womb. If no fertilized ovum is embedded in the endometrium during the endometrial cycle, then the endometrium, or lining of the womb, is shed. This shedding of the lining of the womb presents as bleeding from the womb. Thus, if there is no fertilized ovum, or pregnancy, the shedding of the lining of the womb can occur approximately each month. This is referred to as menstruation, the menses, or a menstrual period.

When the fertilized ovum becomes embedded in the endometrium, the uterine lining is not shed. This continues as a pregnancy.

The human male does not have a uterus. Thus, men do not menstruate or have menstrual periods. This is one of the many reasons why men cannot get pregnant!
It is not an unusual phenomenon for men to pass blood in their semen. This is called hematospermia. This may result from any inflammatory condition of the prostate gland or the seminal vesicle.

One of the most frequent causes of prostate irritation is the ingestion of caffeine. This condition is known as prostatitis. This can also be due to the intake of alcohol or other "blood thinners," such as very spicy foods, infections, or even the act of sexual intercourse itself. This is sometimes seen with no identifiable cause.

Men may pass blood after sex, but men do not menstruate.

37

An impotent man cannot produce a pregnancy.

FACT:

Sperm production and ejaculation are not dependent upon a man's ability to get or maintain an erection. An erection facilitates the transportation of semen.

The semen, containing sperm, can be released with or without an erection. So, if a man is impotent the semen can still be released, thereby causing a pregnancy. It is also possible for the pre-ejaculate to contain enough sperm to cause a pregnancy.

38

Viagra causes heart problems.

FACT:

This myth is based primarily upon misinformation. Viagra contains an ingredient called sildenafil.

Sildenafil can effectively treat chest pains in individuals with heart problems. Many people misconstrue this to mean that sildenafil causes the heart problem.

This medication can result in increased blood flow in small vessels, such as those supplying the penis with blood. This increased blood flow to the penis can aid in getting erections. Before starting on such medication, it is always best to consult a physician. An asymptomatic heart problem may be uncovered. In such cases, the sildenafil (Viagra) should not be blamed for causing the heart problem.

39

Aphrodisiacs are the best form of treatment for impotence.

FACT:

Aphrodisiacs are substances that stimulate or increase one's desire for sex. Interestingly, anything that a person associates with sex can serve as an aphrodisiac for that person. This can take the form of an item of food, an odor, a pill, or indeed other items.

Impotence is the inability to achieve or maintain an erection that is satisfactory for sexual intercourse. Impotence is often a symptom of an underlying medical condition. The successful treatment of impotence may thus depend upon successfully identifying the cause of it. Most cases of impotence are due to an organic or physical reason. Many conditions are known to cause impotence, such as diabetes, hypertension, neurological disorders, pelvic cancers, depression, and many others.

Even if an item, called an aphrodisiac, increases a desire for sex, that item is unlikely to treat the cause of impotence. In fact, the aphrodisiac may even worsen the condition. A person with impotence due to atherosclerosis may identify an egg as an aphrodisiac. Eating eggs may increase the desire for sex but is unlikely to help his atherosclerosis.

The best form of treatment for impotence depends upon establishing the cause of the condition. A urologist is the physician best suited to treat this problem.

40

Lime or lemon juice cuts a man's "courage".

FACT:

The thinking of many individuals is that lemon juice decreases the libido and keeps a man from getting erections. If this were true lemonade would not be so popular!

Lime or lemon juice is good for detoxifying, cleansing the body, and helping to maintain a normal alkalization of the body, but has nothing to do with a man's "courage."

41

If a man had many sexual partners when he was young, he will not be able to perform when he gets older.

FACT:

Sexual performance at any point in time is not an indication of the number of previous sexual partners, in males or females.

The number of sexual partners during youth and adolescence will not determine a man's sexual potency later in life. Many men believe that "running around" in younger years caused them to "slow down" as they get older. There are more important factors influencing older men's performance than the number of women they had sex with during their younger years. These factors include overall state of health, emotional health and even the andropause.

Sexual prowess in an older man is strongly influenced by his state of health. Common causes of sexual dysfunction in older men include diabetes, hypertension, neurological disorders, cardiovascular conditions, medication, drugs, lifestyle, and emotional disorders. His performance is often a reflection of his cardiovascular health.

An often overlooked factor in a man's sexual performance is the andropause. This is the gradual decline in hormones, such as growth hormone and testosterone, as he gets older. These hormones aided his muscular physique, metabolism, and stamina during his younger years. A decrease in libido and performance is common during the andropause.

FEMALES AND SEXUAL MYTHS

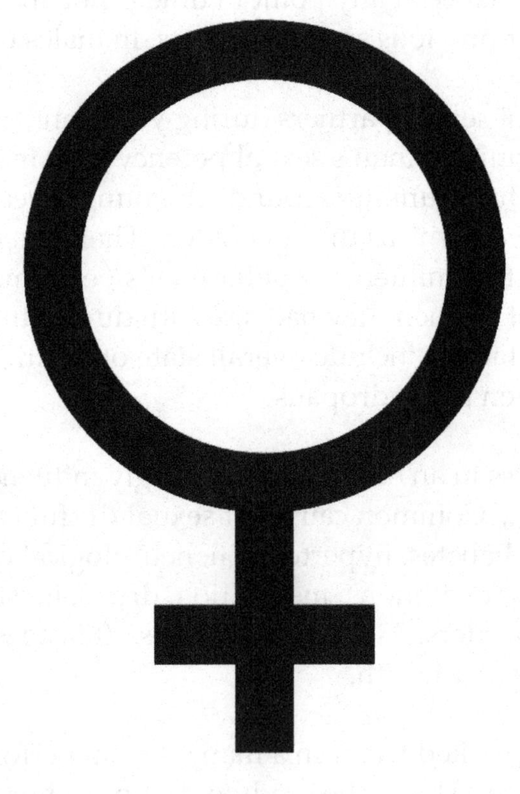

42

Women don't really enjoy sex.

FACT:

Women enjoy sex as much as men do.

Men may equate sexual enjoyment more with vaginal penetration than women do. Women tend to want more cuddling and play time than men, but they want that orgasm too.

I heard a woman say that some folk enjoy a cup of coffee to get going each morning, but she enjoys sex each morning to get her going for the day.

43

Some women don't have a clitoris.

FACT:

The clitoris is more, or less, prominent in some women than in others. A less prominent clitoris does not diminish a woman's enjoyment of sexual intercourse or her ability to achieve an orgasm.

44

When the hymen is broken, she has had sex before.

FACT:

It is not true that only sexual intercourse breaks the hymen. Disruption of the hymen may be due to vigorous exercise, horseback riding, cycling, masturbation, use of tampons, or medical examination.

It should be noted that the presence of the hymen is not proof that no previous sexual contact had been made.

45

Douching is the best way to keep the vagina clean.

FACT:

The vagina is self-cleaning. Douching can be harmful by disturbing the natural bacterial flora balance of the vagina. Furthermore, infection can be spread to the fallopian tubes and ovaries by douching.

If there is a problem with the health of the vagina it is best to consult the appropriate health care provider.

46

A big hand, feet or shoe size in a woman means that she has a big vagina.

FACT:

Not so. Vaginal size is not dependent on the size of body appendages. It may be influenced by such factors as coital frequency, childbirth, pelvic surgery, and vaginal atrophy of aging brought on by hormonal changes.

A book's cover does not always adequately portray its contents. Likewise, a person's appendages do not necessarily portray the characteristics of internal organs.

47

In Chinese women, the vagina lies cross-wise.

FACT:

This is an old, common myth, believed by many men and women. Since my youth, I wondered if this were true, or, indeed, if not, how did the myth get started.

Many people believe that in Chinese females the labia at the vaginal introitus lay horizontally rather than vertically. This is incorrect. There is no evidence that the basic anatomy of humans depends upon race or national origin. There is nothing strange or unusual about pelvic anatomy in Chinese females.

Sorry fellows, you cannot tell a woman's country of origin by what's under her skirt!

48

Every woman has a G-spot.

FACT:

The G-spot was popularized in a book by Ernst Grafenberg in 1982. Since then many have tried to find this erogenous zone in the anterior wall of the vagina. There is no such defined anatomic structure in the vagina.

A few individuals claim to have found the G-spot. Most are still looking for it.

49

A condom can get lost in a woman's body.

FACT:

If a condom slips off during vaginal sex, the condom would be in the vagina, and is retrievable. It would not be expected to enter the uterus because the cervix is normally not sufficiently open for the condom to enter. It would not enter the abdominal cavity either because the cul-de-sac (end of the vagina) is a closed area.

In the case of anal coitus, a dislodged condom is easily retrievable by a health care provider.

50

You can lose your virginity by having a Pap smear done.

FACT:

You are a virgin until you have engaged in sexual intercourse. A doctor's examination or evaluation has nothing to do with your status or loss of virginity.

Your doctor is concerned about your health and wellbeing. Even if the hymen is no longer intact after your examination or evaluation you are still a virgin, if you have not had sex. Having a Pap smear has nothing to do with your virginity.

51

A woman is less of a woman after having a hysterectomy.

FACT:

A hysterectomy is a commonly performed operation. In this procedure, only the womb (uterus) is surgically removed. A woman is just as much a woman after the hysterectomy as she was before the operation. This operation does not change a woman's sexuality and/or femininity. Sexual enjoyment should remain intact after a hysterectomy. She remains as beautiful and attractive as she was prior to her surgery. Of course, she would not be able to bear children because of the removal of the womb.

Some women feel more sexually liberated after the hysterectomy because the procedure has resolved a burdensome problem. Sex is thus more enjoyable for many women. Similarly, a woman of fertile age has no concern about pregnancy after this operation.

Note that an oophorectomy is the removal of the ovaries. This may or may not be done at the time of the hysterectomy. This may also result in hormonal changes in the woman, which could possibly affect her libido.

There are important medical indications for a hysterectomy procedure, including:

- Cancer of the uterus, cervix, ovaries, and fallopian tubes

- Menorrhagia, or heavy menstrual bleeding, severe enough to cause anemia
- Metrorrhagia, heavy blood loss between menstrual periods
- Severe prolapse of the uterus. This is the condition where the pelvic muscles and ligaments are no longer supporting the uterus. The uterus falls into the vagina and may protrude outside of the vagina.
- Chronic pelvic pain, such as in the condition known as endometriosis.
- Fibroids, none cancerous tumors of the uterus, causing compromise of other organs, like the bowels and urinary bladder.

52

Women don't like to give oral sex.

FACT:

Not true. Oral sex wouldn't be so popular if women didn't like, and enjoy, it.

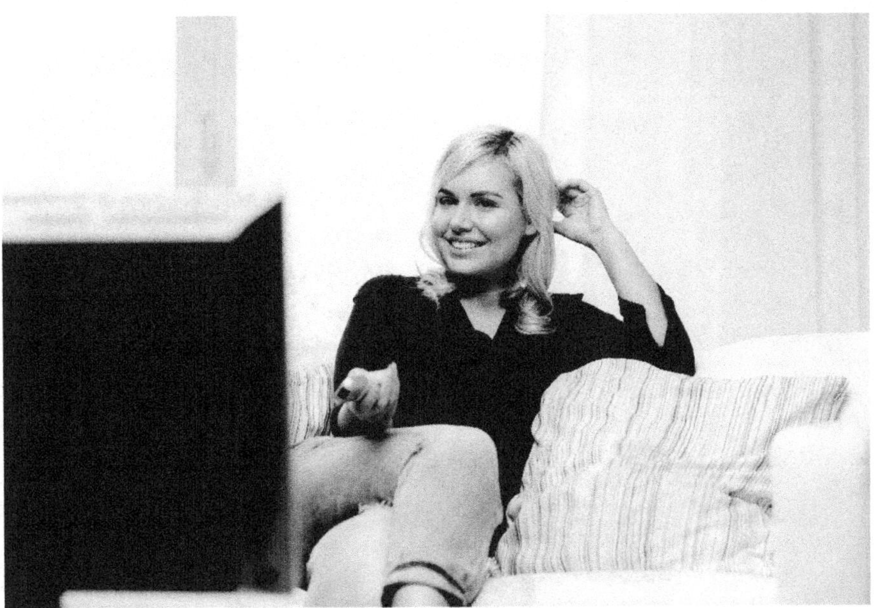

53

Women don't like pornography or dirty sex.

FACT:

Women like this stuff just like men do.

Men do not have a monopoly on pornography. Women fantasize as much as men do. Women are also susceptible to pornography addiction.

Keep in mind, erotic paraphernalia and clothing for females is big, big business.

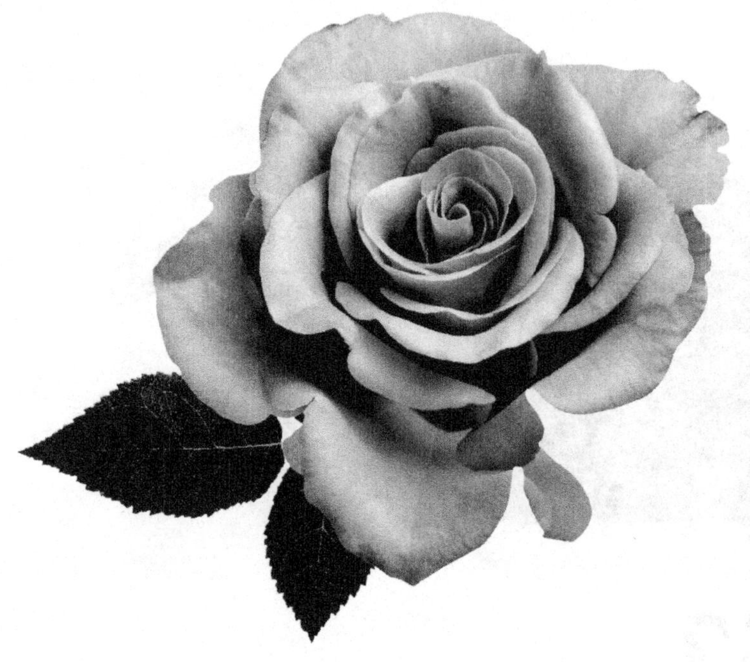

54

A woman is not fully a woman if she can't get pregnant.

FACT:

There are many possible reasons why a woman may not be able to become pregnant. Pregnancy is not a requirement for female maturation. Some women make personal, conscious decisions not to get pregnant, for whatever reasons they choose.

Some reasons for female non-fertility include:

- Congenital anomalies. These may include chromosomal abnormalities and physical defects like incompletely developed or missing organs.
- Postmenopausal state. The ovaries no longer produce eggs.
- Hormonal imbalances. Not only must hormones be present, but they must be present in specific ratios to each other. A hormone level too high or too low can interfere with normal functioning of some tissues or organs.
- Medication. Many medications can interfere with, or prevent pregnancy. An example of this is the birth control pill.
- Implant devises. These include the IUD's (intrauterine devices)
- Pelvic surgery. Any surgery in the pelvic region has the potential of affecting the reproductive system.
- Pelvic infections. Pelvic infections can affect the female reproductive system. For example, gonorrhea can cause inflammation and obstruction of the fallopian tubes, rendering a woman infertile.
- Pelvic trauma
- Certain medical conditions
- Sexual abstinence
- Idiopathic (Unknown). Many women appear to be normal in every respect but do not get pregnant. Nature has the upper hand in many of these cases.

55

Don't drink out of a bottle during pregnancy. This would cause the baby to be strangled.

FACT:

Strangling refers to asphyxiation, or difficulty in breathing. Certainly, the unborn child would not have this problem. The first breath is taken after the baby is delivered. Difficulty breathing at that time is likely due to immaturity of the respiratory structures. Cystic fibrosis, a genetic disorder, can also cause difficulties in breathing for the newborn child. Drinking from a bottle, or any other container, would have no effect on a developing baby. Mom's choice of drink container also has nothing to do with finding the umbilical cord around the baby's neck at delivery, and would not cause strangling in the newborn.

The contents of the bottle may affect both mother and child. For example, alcohol can directly affect a pregnant uterus. So, beware of what you are drinking during pregnancy.

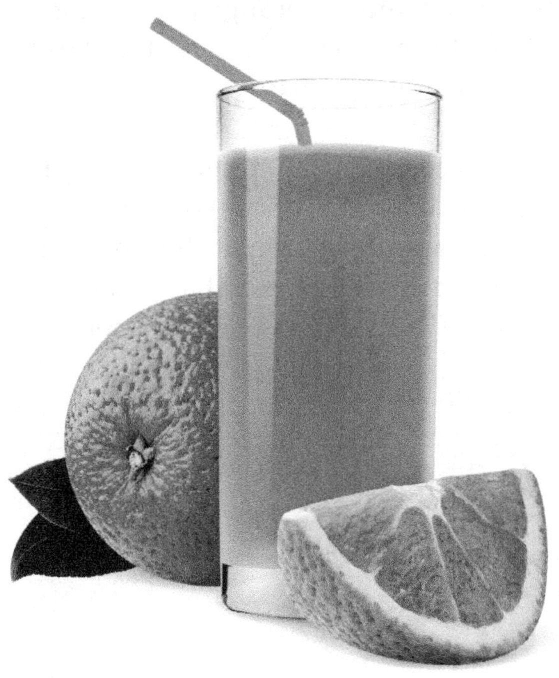

56

Drinking a lot of orange juice during pregnancy produces a pretty baby.

FACT:

If this were true, the states of Florida and California would be full of pretty people. Orange juice has no known human phenotypic genetic activity. Orange juice is good stuff but it cannot claim this kind of credit.

Despite its nutritional contents, orange juice is not known for producing DNA or chromosomal changes that affect the physical attributes of a fetus or baby.

Mom and dad must accept responsibility for the physical attributes of their child. Orange juice will not change the contributions of the parents, as seen in their baby. Even pure citric acid won't help after conception has taken place. A baby's looks are sealed at the time of conception.

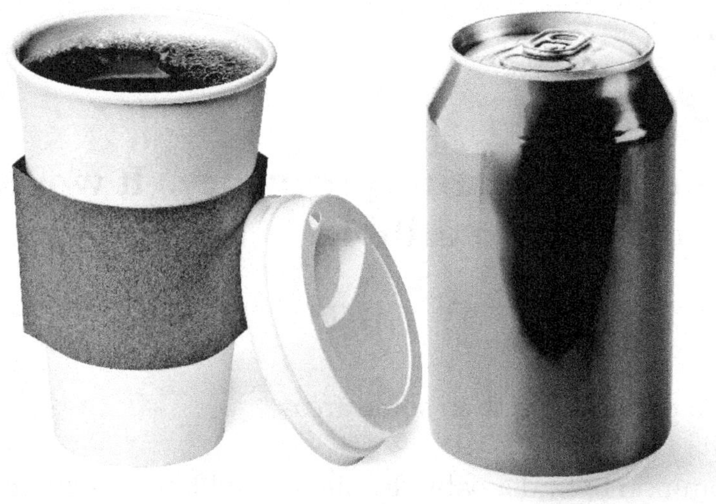

57

If a pregnant woman drinks a lot of coffee or Coca Cola her baby would be dark.

FACT:

This myth appears to have the slightest bit of logic in it. However, it is simply not true. These drinks contain no genetic melanin, the stuff that determines skin color. They can't darken anything during or after conception. Mommy must check out her own skin hues or that of daddy's.

Incidentally, daddy's intake of dark drinks won't contribute to the baby's melanin count either. Daddy and Mommy's genetics are the sole determinants of the baby's skin hues.

58

Don't eat okra during pregnancy. It would cause the baby to dribble.

FACT:

This is a common myth in some areas.

It is common to find a baby drooling, dribbling or salivating. Control of such dribbling may require coordination of multiple systems and functions in the baby's body. A baby's nervous and muscular systems are not fully developed or fully functional at birth. This includes brain development.

Give the baby time to develop!

Eating okra during pregnancy will not negatively influence the baby's development. Okra is a nutritious vegetable and may be the very thing that the mother needs, especially if she is anemic. Okra contains many nutrients including minerals like calcium, iron, copper, selenium, magnesium, manganese and zinc, complex vitamins such as A, C, and K together with the all-important B vitamin, which contains folate for protecting the baby's developing spine and spinal cord, and other good stuff like anti-oxidants, fiber, and mucilage.

59

Hanging clothes on a high line during pregnancy would cause the baby's neck to pop.

FACT:

This myth suggests that over-reaching during pregnancy would affect the physical integrity of the baby's musculoskeletal systems. Not true at all. Activities of the mother's extremities during pregnancy do not determine what happens to the baby's neck.

An injury to the baby's neck can occur during delivery, especially in a difficult or complicated delivery. Even so, this is not a common occurrence.

60

If a woman gets pregnant by a drunk man, the baby would be born drunk.

FACT:

When a man's liver metabolizes alcohol, his sperm are not influenced. Imagine a drunken sperm trying to find its way into and out of the vagina, through the cervix, through the uterus and out into the fallopian tube. If it makes it through this journey, then the drunken sperm finds the egg and fertilizes it.

If this were true, the king of beers could also be an army general!

Alcohol ingestion by a woman can affect the pregnant uterus. However, daddy's drink before impregnation won't affect her uterus at all, let alone nine months later.

61

Women who have only one breast are freaks. Men don't enjoy having sex with them.

FACT:

Many men are sexually turned on by breasts, boobs, and cleavage.

Two breasts may be necessary for cleavage but are not necessary for successful sexual activity. Good sex can occur without a woman baring, or exposing, her chest.

A mastectomy is the surgical removal of the breast. There is nothing freaky about the woman who undergoes a mastectomy, for whatever reason. This procedure is often done to protect a woman from the dreaded disease of breast cancer. The operation is performed about 50,000 times a year in the United States.

Some women who have a mastectomy elect to have reconstructive surgery where implants are placed under the skin to simulate the appearance of a normal breast. Other women have autologous reconstruction done, using her skin, muscle, and fat tissue for breast reconstruction. Many women use a breast prosthesis in a fitted bra. These prostheses are properly fitted by size and color to meet the woman's expectations and desires.

There are women who simply accept the fact that the breast, and cancer, are gone. They are happy to be alive and well, and move on with their lives. Of course, there are some women who need all of the encouragement and support that they can get.

A man who thinks of a woman with one breast as a freak probably needs to revamp his own thinking of women and educate himself on the medical challenges which the woman has faced. He should consider ways that he can help such a woman maintain her own sense of civility and self-esteem.

62

A woman's sex life ends at menopause.

FACT:

At menopause, a woman's body undergoes hormonal and physiologic changes. The ovaries no longer produce eggs; thus, pregnancy can no longer occur. Although her reproductive life ends, her sex life may continue for many more years.

Estrogen and progesterone hormone production dramatically decrease at this time. These changes affect women differently. Some women experience vaginal dryness, resulting in uncomfortable sex. Their libido may also decrease. Some women however, experience no such changes.

A gynecologist can assist a woman if she experiences untoward effects at the menopause, so that she can continue to have an enjoyable sex life.

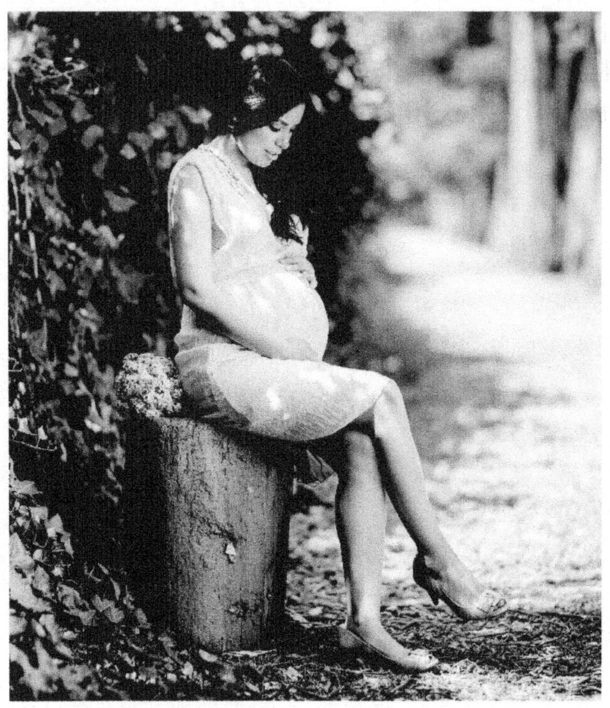

63

Don't cross your legs in pregnancy because the umbilical cord would tangle.

FACT:

The umbilical cord is the conduit that attaches the developing fetus to the placenta, the tissue in the womb from which the fetus gets its oxygen, nutrients, etc. The umbilical cord is also known as the navel string or birth cord. Its Latin name is funiculus umbilicus. At the time of delivery, the umbilical cord is clamped and cut. The stump is left attached to the baby. It atrophies and falls off a few days later.

During pregnancy one of two entanglements of the cord is likely to occur. An entanglement called a nuchal cord or nuchal loops occurs in about a quarter of all babies. The nuchal cord is one that is wrapped around the baby's neck at delivery. This is usually not serious, and usually does not interfere with the baby's blood supply. It doesn't cause suffocation of the baby because the baby does not start breathing on its own until the cord is severed at delivery. The other entanglement is known as umbilical cord knots. These occur in a few cases, about 1 out of 100 deliveries. These umbilical knots can form during pregnancy by movements of the developing baby or even during delivery of the baby. These are sometimes seen in cases of identical twins.

Obstetricians are always alert to these entanglements and manage them very well.

Fortunately, a pregnant woman's legs have nothing to do with the umbilical cord of her developing baby. The safety of her baby will not depend upon whether her legs are crossed or not during her pregnancy.

64

If a pregnant woman holds her arms above her head, the umbilical cord can get wrapped around the baby's neck.

FACT:

It is not unusual for the umbilical cord to be wrapped around the baby's neck. In fact, this reportedly occurs in about 25% of births. This occurrence is referred to as a nuchal cord or nuchal loops.

The mother's physical activities are not known to be associated with nuchal cords. These nuchal cords are known to be due to movement of the baby in the amniotic fluid prior to birth.

The position of a pregnant woman's arms or legs have nothing to do with the occurrence of nuchal cords.

65

If a pregnant woman points at a man, the baby would be born looking like the man.

FACT:

Oh, what a myth! This can only be true if she points at the man for whom she is pregnant.

The physical characteristics of the baby are determined by the genetic material contained in the father's sperm and the mother's egg at the time of conception. No physical drills by mom or dad during pregnancy will alter the DNA of a developing baby.

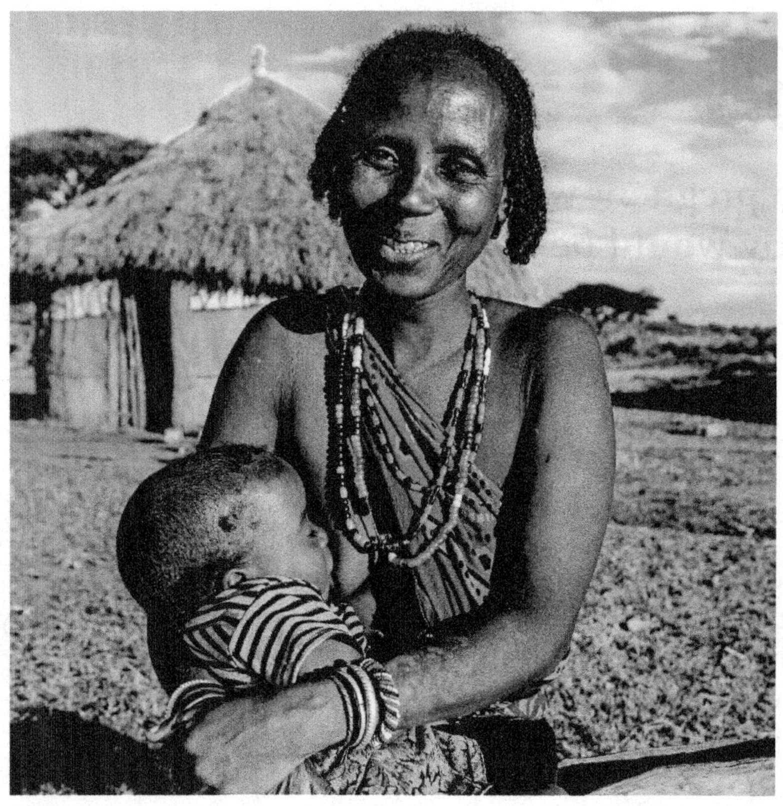

66

If you don't have mommy, you can suck granny.

FACT:

There is widespread belief that if the nursing mother is not available, the grandmother can breast feed the baby. Granny may provide comfort for the baby and even have a "good feeling" doing so, but no granny milk is likely to be forth coming.

Unless granny has also recently given birth it is unlikely that she will produce milk on demand. Chances are that granny's alveoli and ducts (milk producers) have already atrophied (dried up).

Normal breast milk production requires the proper release and balance of hormones such as prolactin, oxytocin, progesterone, and estrogen. Granny had her day!

67

When a woman says no to sex she actually means yes.

FACT:

While this may be true in a specific situation, it is best to take a woman "at her word."

Going forward with sex when a person says NO means sexual assault. Be aware that a woman can say NO without using the word "NO." Even a gesture can mean NO. She may shake her head, wave a finger, cross her legs, turn her back, refuse to disrobe or simply say "not now," "not here," or "not this time."

68

Vaginal penetration is necessary to produce a pregnancy.

FACT:

Certainly not. Sperms produce pregnancy, not penile penetration. Penile penetration can occur all day but no pregnancy can occur without the production of sperm. This is evidenced by the fact that an azospermic male can have sex but cannot produce a pregnancy. After a vasectomy, erections are normal but no pregnancy occurs. On the other hand, sperm can be produced and find their way into the vagina without penile penetration of the vagina. In terms of pregnancy, this is the danger of unprotected foreplay, and after play as well. I have heard of girls claiming to have become pregnant all by themselves because they were never "penetrated."

Some think that ejaculation must occur within the vagina for pregnancy to occur. This is not accurate. This is one of the reasons that "pulling out" is so unreliable for preventing pregnancy. It is also well known that the pre-ejaculate may contain sperm, and if this occurs near the vagina, bingo!

69

Women bring sexual abuse upon themselves.

FACT:

This myth is suggestive of a perpetrator blaming the victim.

Women are often blamed for being sexy, seductive, hot, provocative, drunk or whatever. Regardless of how women present themselves a perpetrator of abuse has the responsibility of self-control. When a person loses control of himself he is subject to civil, criminal, and even religious disobedience. The consequences of such disobedience depends upon the mentality of the disobedient.

Abuse may occur in the form of:

- Verbal abuse
- Physical abuse
- Sexual abuse - violent or nonviolent
- Intimidation
- Threats or acts of violence
- Deprivation of privileges
- Isolation

Blaming others does not release anyone from acts of abuse. There are many instances where a man was seduced, provoked, lied against, and even attacked, but did not respond in an abusive manner.

CONTRACEPTION AND SEXUAL MYTHS

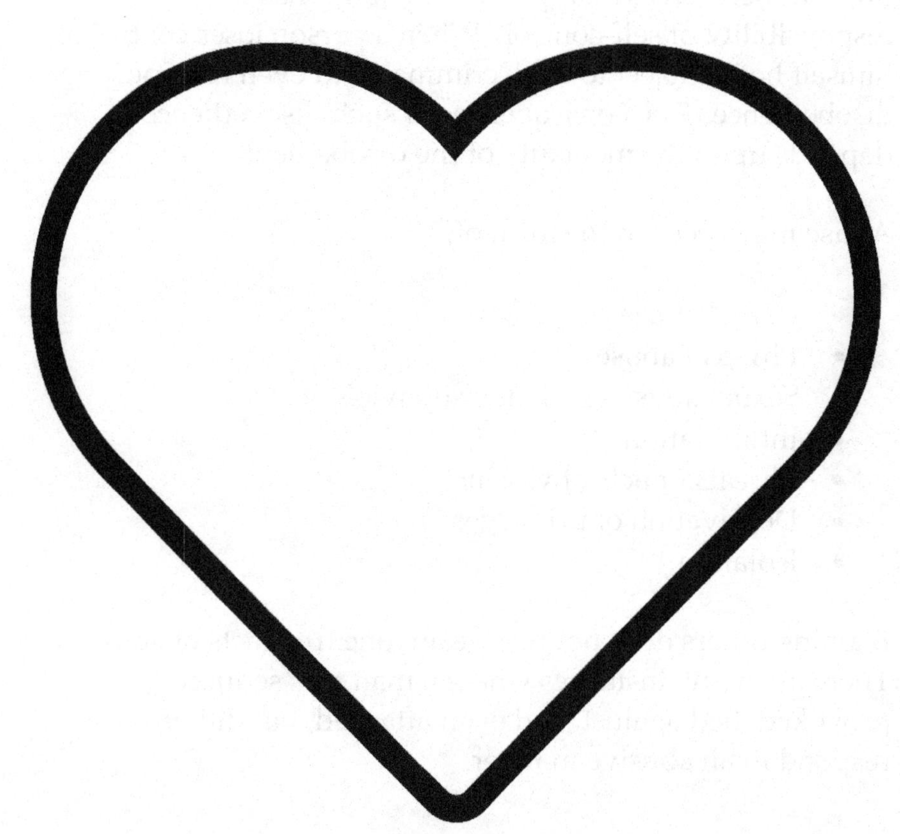

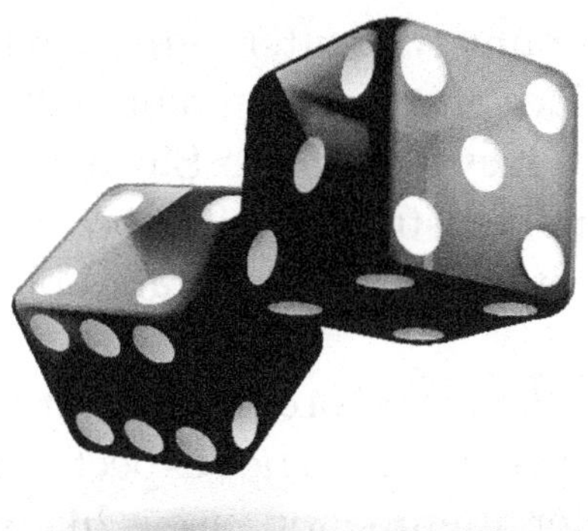

70

You can't get pregnant the first time you have sex.

FACT:

Don't bet on it.

Pregnancy can occur anytime unprotected sexual intercourse takes place in fertile females. If the male is producing sperm and the female is ovulating, pregnancy can occur. Sperm and eggs believe in love at first sight too.

Sperm and eggs are not good at keeping records of when or how many times a couple has sex. Pregnancy requires only one intercourse, whether it is the first or last time.

Pregnancy can occur any time after ovulation begins. If intercourse takes place after ovulation but before the start of menstruation, pregnancy is possible. Since ovulation occurs fourteen days before menstruation, it is possible for pregnancy to occur before the first menstruation takes place.

If the first sexual contact is before the start of ovulation and menstruation, then pregnancy is not expected to occur. The first sexual encounter after menopause is likewise not expected to result in a pregnancy.

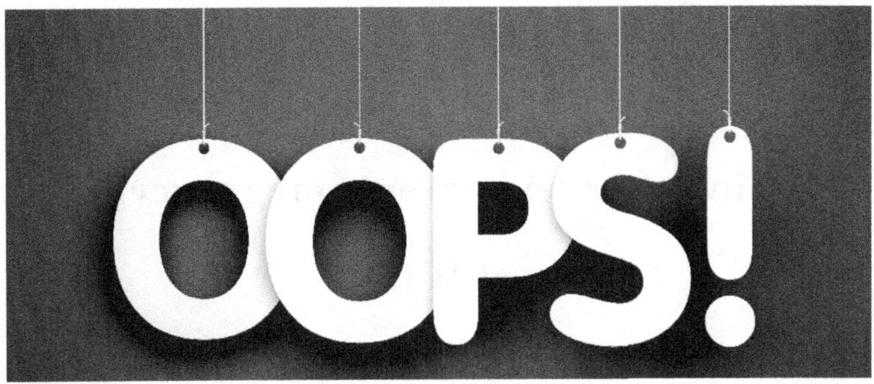

71

I won't get pregnant if he pulls out.

FACT:

This is known as coitus interruptus. Pulling out may or may not work. Chances are that it won't work.

There is no way to tell when it is the right moment to withdraw. Furthermore, it may be psychologically difficult to withdraw even if you intend to. Sometimes it is just plain hard to stop a good thing!

As in basketball, a man may dribble before he shoots. This pre-ejaculate may contain enough sperm to produce a pregnancy. Remember that only one sperm is needed to produce a pregnancy. Even if ejaculation takes place outside of the vagina, sperm can swim back inside. Those guys know where to go.

Orgasm is not required for pregnancy to occur. So, while waiting for orgasm the work of producing a pregnancy may have already been done.

72

Douching after sex prevents pregnancy.

FACT:

This is unlikely.

Sperm can move fast enough to be beyond the reach of the douche by the time douching takes place.

Some individuals believe that douching with coca cola would be effective. Douching with coke can be harmful to vaginal tissue and is not a good idea.

73

The pill works 100% of the time.

FACT:

Only abstinence is 100%, and abstinence must mean no physical or sexual contact.   When taken properly the pill is very effective as a means of contraception.

Remember that if an occurrence is one in a million and you are that one, the others don't count!

74

Using another person's birth control pill will work just as well.

FACT:

A birth control pill is a prescribed medication.

A prescription is a physician's order for a specific person, to be used as ordered, in the amount prescribed, for the period of time as ordered by the prescribing physician. Birth control pills contain powerful hormones. The appropriate health care provider must monitor the effects of this medication.

Never take another person's prescribed medication. Many factors are considered in determining a prescription such as allergies, sensitivities, previous and present medication, age, medical history, availability of medicines, possible reactions with other medication, etc. Taking another person's medication can have possible serious side effects.
Taking any medication haphazardly can be dangerous.

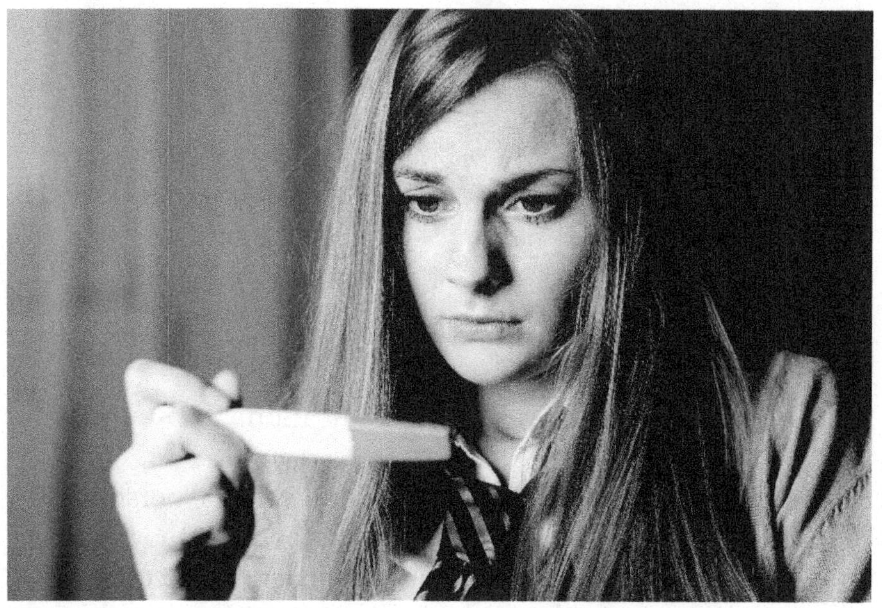

75

Birth control pills work for men also.

FACT:

Birth control pills, to date, are for females only.

I saw an interesting case of lost libido in a young man. I was a bit puzzled until I discovered that he was taking the birth control pill instead of his wife.

Birth control pills are designed to work on the female reproductive system and work by regulating menstruation by controlling ovulation.

76

Birth control pills make you gain weight.

FACT:

There is no scientific evidence for this. Weight gain and obesity are more likely due to caloric intake rather than taking a birth control pill. There may be some increase in fluid retention in some individuals but overall weight gain is likely to be due to other factors.

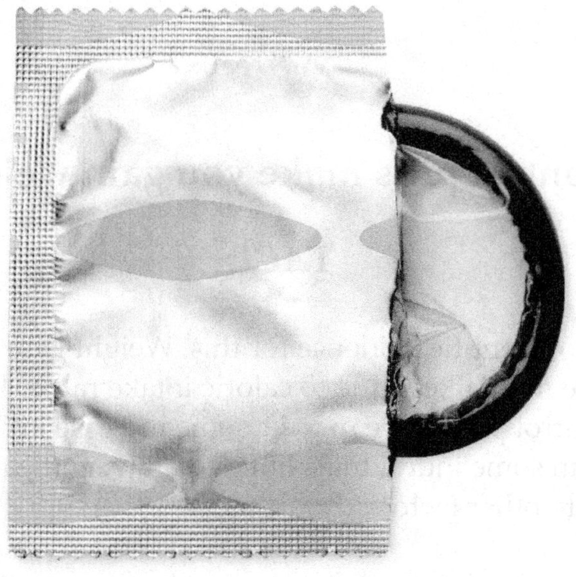

77

A condom guarantees safety against pregnancy.

FACT:

Condoms are notoriously unreliable for protection against pregnancy. They are often ill fitting, rupture, perforate easily, or slip off. Sometimes they are even deliberately taken off. Want to make a mint? Just design a well-fitting, puncture proof condom that stays put!

78

Wearing two condoms double the protection against pregnancy.

FACT:

Wearing two condoms will only give you a false sense of security. In fact, the friction between the condoms would increase the chances of rupture in one of them.
In this case two is not better than one.

79

Condoms are 100% safe.

FACT:

Condoms are not fool proof even when used properly. Many men (and women) can attest to the fact that condoms cannot give 100% guarantee against pregnancy. Why? Because no one has designed a condom that won't slip off or one that is puncture proof. Wearing a condom may reduce the incidence of some STD'S but this is not guaranteed in any individual case either.

Sometimes a condom is worn because of certain "effects," like the ribbed, knotted, glow in the dark, or flavored variety. These are no safer than the regular condoms.

80

A nursing woman can't get pregnant.

FACT:

Many women have gone to their obstetrician for a postnatal visit and were told that they are pregnant-------again. Ovulation may be postponed while breasts feeding but it can occur, thus pregnancy is still possible.

81

You can't get pregnant during your period.

FACT:

This has some logic to it. Implantation of the ovum (fertilized egg) is unlikely during menstruation.

A short or irregular cycle may allow pregnancy to possibly occur because the sperm can survive for several days.

Avoiding a pregnancy means taking protective measures at all times.

82

If there is penile penetration but no ejaculation, pregnancy won't occur.

FACT:

Don't bet on it.

Sperm may be present in the pre-ejaculate fluid, enough to produce a pregnancy. Only one sperm is needed to fertilize the egg for pregnancy.

A rip-roaring orgasm is not necessary for ejaculation to occur either. A less dramatic ejaculation may occur unnoticed. Sperm may also be released unnoticed.

Any penile penetration of the vagina in an unprotected fertile female runs the risk of pregnancy. This is why coitus interruptus is so unreliable for preventing pregnancy.

Withdrawal may occur after the deed has been done! Women are known to say, "But, he didn't discharge in me." She may not have been aware of his "discharge" but she may well have to "discharge" the duties of her pregnancy and that of a mother.

83

You can't get pregnant having sex standing up.

FACT:

Sperm are not good judges of coital positions. They can swim uphill or downhill. Coital position is not usually the determining factor in getting pregnant.

Pregnancy can occur whether you are upright, upside down, standing, sitting, bending over, lying down, or hanging from a rafter!

Also, note that pregnancy can occur whether you are clothed or naked.

84

You can't get pregnant if you don't have an orgasm.

FACT:

An orgasm, in a male or female, is not required for pregnancy.

Many women, about 50%, don't experience regular orgasms. Ovulation is not dependent upon what happens during intercourse. If women have sex during their fertile period, then pregnancy is possible, whether they enjoyed intercourse or not.

Orgasm in men is also not required for pregnancy. Sperm can be released with or without an orgasm. Sperm can be found in the pre-ejaculate fluid and these can also produce a pregnancy.

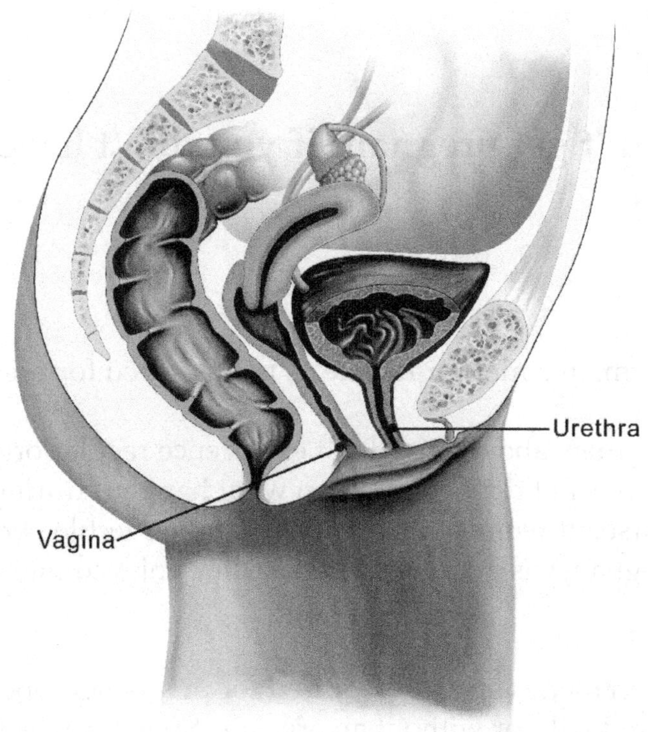

85

Urinating after sex prevents pregnancy.

FACT:

It is surprising how many women believe this popular myth. Many women believe that if they urinate immediately after sex, they will get rid of the ejaculate and sperm. Urinating after sex will only give a woman a false sense of security.

The urinary and reproductive systems are separate systems in females. Sperm entering the reproductive tract in the female do not ordinarily enter the urinary tract. So, post coital voiding of urine won't wash out the female reproductive tract.

When the ejaculate, and sperm, enter the vagina, the sperm traverses the cervix, then on through the uterus on its way to the fallopian tube. No amount of urination will interrupt that journey, especially after passing through the gateway of the cervix!

86

It's the girl's responsibility not to get pregnant.

FACT:

Pregnancy results from sexual intercourse between two people, except in cases of artificial insemination. Both individuals have the responsibility of protecting against an unwanted pregnancy. There are multiple ways of preventing an unwanted pregnancy for men and women. Some techniques are intended for immediate protection, others are intended for long term protection.

Male methods of contraception include use of the condom, a vasectomy, and the mainly unreliable rhythm and coitus interruptus methods. Newer methods under development include intra-vas deferens devices and hormone regulation, that is, a male version of "the contraceptive pill."

Female methods of contraception include the rhythm method, birth control pills, intrauterine devices, cervical caps, spermicide gels and foams, tubal ligation, hormonal patches and injections, and cervical rings.

The only certain and proven method of contraception for males and females is abstinence! Should pregnancy occur, both sexual partners will have the responsibility of caring for the child.

87

A woman cannot get pregnant during a rape. Her body has protective mechanisms that will prevent the pregnancy.

FACT:

This myth is simply that, a myth.

This idea stems from the belief that the stress of a rape would shut down the reproductive processes during the rape.

We know that acute stress can produce physiologic consequences. These consequences may be manifested as tears and crying, sweating, trembling, skin rashes, screaming or quietness, abdominal pain, heart palpitations, headaches, visual disturbances, elevated blood sugar levels, nervousness, bedwetting, urinary and fecal incontinence and even paralysis.

The fact that while there may be physiologic changes in a woman's body during a rape, there is no guarantee that sperm from the rapist and a released egg from the victim would not undergo fertilization. This is evidenced by the many documented cases of pregnancies resulting from rape.

88

If a pregnant woman looks or laughs at a crippled person, the baby would be born with the infirmity of the crippled person.

FACT:

The nervous and musculoskeletal system in the fetus are not influenced by who the mother looks at or interacts with. There is no direct connection between these developing systems and the outside world.

Deficiencies in nutritional factors may play a role in the child's development.   For example, a lack of folate may influence the normal development of the spinal column in the fetus. This would have nothing to do with who the pregnant mother interacts with, whether they are crippled or not.
Other macronutrients and micronutrients are crucial in the normal development of the fetus. Some of these include proteins, fats, calcium, phosphorus, zinc, vitamin D, vitamin C and many more.

Men and women with varying infirmities are known to produce normal children. Pregnant nurses, and other healthcare workers, look at the infirm every day, with no effects on their unborn children.

89

Don't scratch during pregnancy. It will mark the baby where the mother scratched.

FACT:

This myth is often offered as an explanation for a baby's "birth mark."

A birth mark is also known by many other names including:

- Angel kiss
- Café au lait spot
- Devil's mark
- Hemangiomas
- Mongolian spot
- Nevi
- Port wine stain
- Salmon patches
- Stalk mark
- Strawberry mark
- Stork bite

A birth mark can appear in any location on the body and vary in size or appearance. There are about as many explanations for birth marks as there are pregnancies around. These explanations range anywhere from a result of looking at another person's birth mark, to the result of an injury during one's past life on earth. It is believed by many that scratching during pregnancy causes the baby to be marked where the mother scratched. Some think that the mark results from a frightening episode during pregnancy.

The fact is that the cause of birth marks is still unknown but they have nothing to do with what happened to a mother's skin during pregnancy.

There are birth marks known as hemangiomas. These are vascular malformations, that is, clusters of tiny blood vessels beneath the skin. Some hemangiomas will resolve over time, some will not. It is always best to have a proper medical evaluation and seek advice if there are any questions about the safety of a birth mark in an infant.

SEXUAL INTERCOURSE AND SEXUAL MYTHS

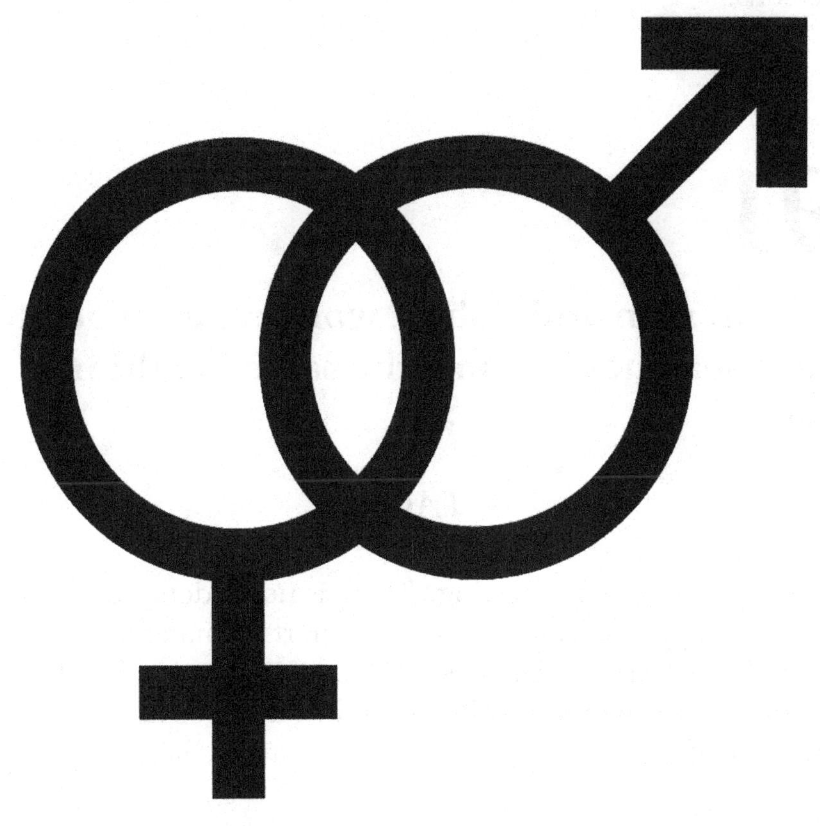

90

Elderly persons should not engage in sex.

FACT:

Age is not the determining factor in sexual activity. One's overall medical, mental, and physical status are likely to be more important. Abraham and Sarah proved that sex in old age can be meaningful. Interestingly, sexually active individuals generally live longer than non-sexually active persons.

91

If a tall man and a short woman get in bed to have sex, they become the same height in bed.

FACT:

This myth is quite interesting. There is no evidence to show that this happens. A tall man and a short woman may be sexually compatible! There is no change in physical height in the man or the woman while in bed or during sexual intercourse.

Sexual compatibility occurs between tall, short, fat, skinny, pretty, and not so pretty people.

92

Happy couples always have good sex.

FACT:

This suggests that a happily married couple almost always has tremendous sex. This may be true but not necessarily so. A wife or husband may have a condition that impacts the frequency and even the performance of sex, yet still be happily married.

There may be a subtle suggestion that happy couples always have spontaneous sex. Of course, spontaneous sex is expected to be "good sex." The anticipation of planned sex, on the other hand, makes for good sex as well.

93

Good sex produces pretty girls and handsome sons.

FACT:

Physical characteristics are genetically determined. Sexual performance has nothing to do with genes, and gene expression, except as a means of passing them on to offspring. Good sex won't change ugly genes into pretty ones, or vice versa. Two short, chubby people having sex won't produce a tall handsome son. Miss World and Mr. Universe are not likely to have the ugliest baby in the neighborhood either. Sexual partners do not participate in gene selection during sex. Good sex, or bad sex, is only what it says.

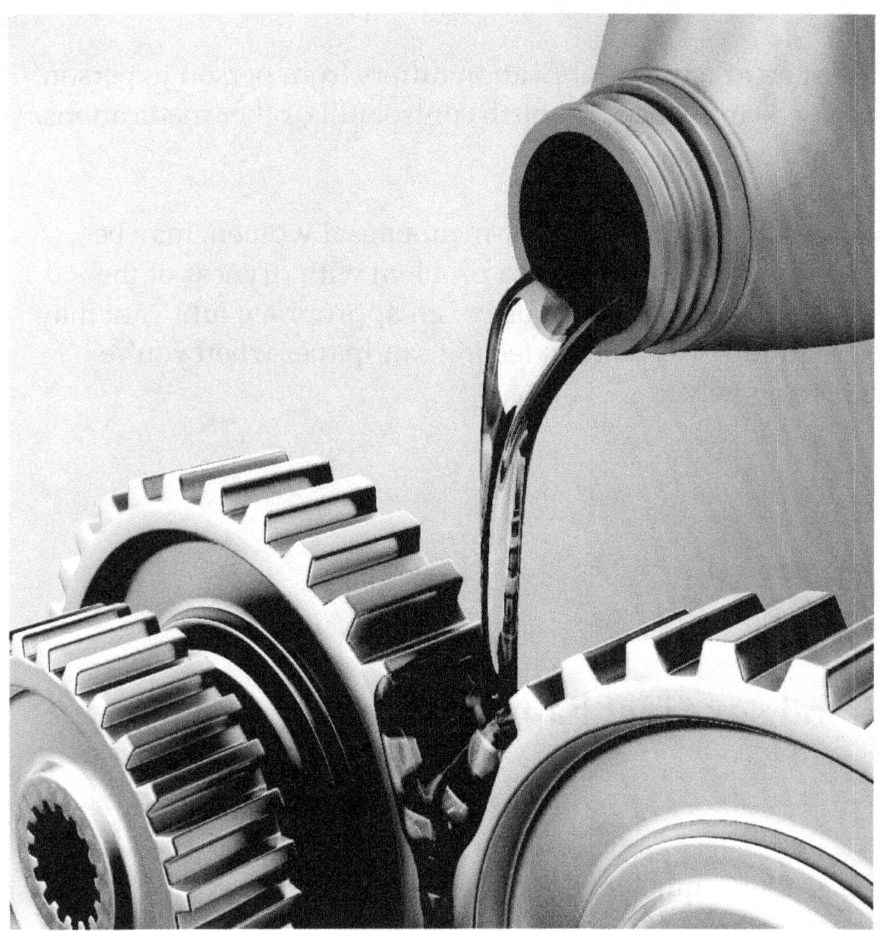

94

If you're really aroused, you shouldn't need any additional lubricant.

FACT:

This may be true for some individuals but not everyone. The amount of lubrication at the start of intercourse may also diminish during sex.

The state of natural lubrication differs from person to person. It may be influenced by birth control pills, other medications, hormones, and even age.

Some individuals, e.g., post-menopausal women, may be sexually aroused but have a problem with dryness of the sexual tissues. Judicious use of an appropriate lubricant may be required. No point in feeling sandpaper when you're expecting velvet.

95

Good sex "just happens".

FACT:

Other than a quickie, a one night stand, good sex won't just happen.

Good sex is an achievement, and it does not happen every time intercourse takes place. Components of good sex include compatibility, desire, intimacy, communication, tolerance, and other such virtues.

96

Sex is a failure if there is no orgasm.

FACT:

An orgasm is not required to have good sex.

Good sex is achieved through closeness, intimacy, communication, tolerance, etc. Some individuals never experience orgasm, but enjoy sex. Only about fifty percent of women have orgasms yet they still find sex to be enjoyable.

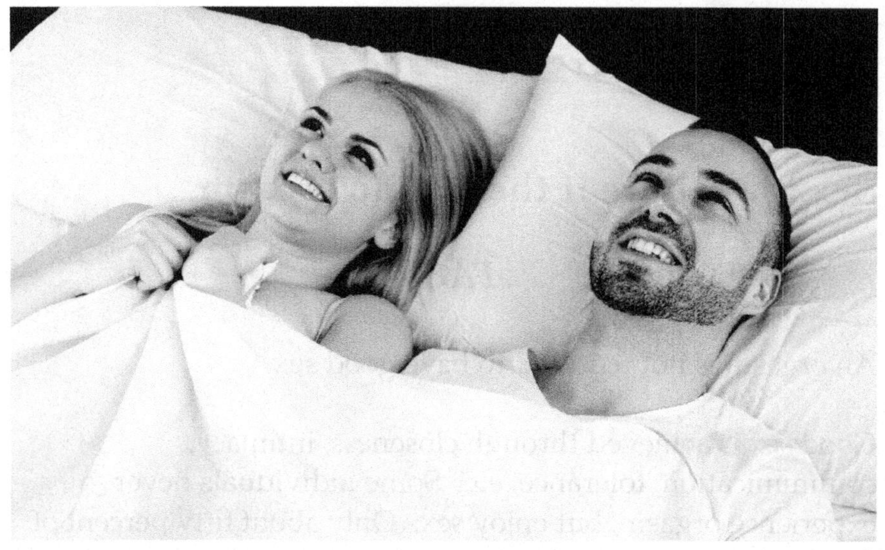

97

A woman must orgasm to enjoy sex.

FACT:

The orgasm may be the peak of sexual enjoyment during intercourse. Only 50% of women reach this peak. This is not to say that only 50% of women enjoy sex. It is not necessary to reach this peak to enjoy sex. The orgasm is not necessary to enjoy sex nor is it necessary for pregnancy to occur.

98

All orgasms are explosive.

FACT:

Orgasms are not always explosive. The orgasm differs from person to person, and from one orgasm to another. The intensity of an orgasm may be anywhere between mild and hardly noticeable, to ecstatically explosive.

The intensity of the orgasm does not determine the enjoyment of sex. In any given situation, the warmth of intimacy, opportunity for close communication, recognition of compatibility, etc., may overshadow the importance of a "great" orgasm.

If the object of intercourse is only to achieve an explosive orgasm, this may be considered a rather selfish approach to sex.

99

The only way for a woman to have an orgasm is through sexual intercourse.

FACT:

Sexual intercourse is a great way for a woman to have an orgasm but it is not the only way.

Clitoral stimulation promotes orgasms in the female. There are numerous ways of stimulating the clitoris, by sexual intercourse, manually, orally and with various paraphernalia, etc.

Some females have orgasms by viewing erotic materials, fantasizing, as well as through close physical contact without sexual intercourse.

100

Simultaneous orgasm is necessary for good sex.

FACT:

Good sex can be enjoyed with or without orgasm. Simultaneous orgasms are good when they occur, but this is not always the case.

Fifty percent of women don't have orgasms but enjoy sex nevertheless. Men do not always have orgasms either, but can still enjoy the closeness and intimacy of sex.

101

All women are multi-orgasmic.

FACT:

Not true.

Only 50% of women have orgasms. It is estimated that about 30% of women have multiple orgasms and 10% have multiple orgasms on a regular basis.

When a male has an orgasm, there is a period of time during which he will not have another orgasm. This is known as the refractory period. Females do not have a refractory period, as in males. Thus, females are physiologically capable of rapid and repeated orgasms.

102

Females ejaculate at orgasm.

FACT:

Ejaculation is a male event. The liquid of semen is produced by the prostate gland and the seminal vesicle. Females do not have prostates or seminal vesicles, and do not produce seminal fluid.

The seminal fluid is an important transport medium for sperm. It provides nutrition for the sperm. Since sperm production is a male function there is no need for the female to produce seminal fluid.

There is a corollary event in females where increased vaginal lubrication occurs at orgasm. Some individuals may mistakenly take this for an ejaculation in the female.

103

You can't tell when a woman is reaching orgasm.

FACT:

Many women do not have slam dunk orgasms. They do, however, enjoy sexual intercourse. The orgasm may be anything from mild to explosively ecstatic. A woman once said that after a great event she had to buy a new bed. It was that great! Another woman said that she had to buy a new dining table after a great sex event!

The male partner may not always know that the woman has reached her peak. However, there are signs of orgasm in the female.

These signs may include the following:

- Acceleration in breathing and heartbeat. Interestingly, some individuals may breathe more slowly
- Flushing of the skin
- The clitoris becomes more erect, and in some women very erect
- The breast nipples become more sensitive
- Increase in vaginal secretions and lubrication
- Rhythmic contraction of the vagina
- Many women become more verbal and expressive

104

A man cannot fake an orgasm.

FACT:

Anyone can fake almost anything. A good actor can put on a good act.

There are recognizable signs of orgasm in the male.

These signs include the following:

- Flushing of the skin
- Acceleration in breathing and heart beat
- Pre-ejaculation may occur
- Contraction of pelvic muscles
- Ejection of semen
- Detumescence of the penis after ejaculation (loss of erection)
- Start of the refractory period. This is the period of time after ejaculation during which a man cannot ejaculate again.

105

Deep vaginal penetration is more sensual for females.

FACT:

Some females enjoy deep thrusting. Others don't. Deep penetration is not always necessary for sexual enjoyment. Nerve endings in the vaginal area are concentrated in the lips and outer areas of the vagina. These are the more sensitive areas. The clitoris is certainly not tucked away deep in the vagina. It is strategically located above the vaginal introitus. Yet, it is the anatomic structure that many women find most excitable.

106

The hymen is always destroyed at the first intercourse.

FACT:

Not necessarily. The hymen is a web of tissue at the vaginal introitus (entrance) in the sexually inactive female. In some females, the hymen may be thick or thin. In others, it may be nearly nonexistent. This tissue may be easily torn or it may be resistant.

The effect of the first intercourse on the hymen varies a lot, depending upon the condition of the hymen. It is not unusual that more than one attempt at intercourse is necessary to completely interrupt the hymen. So, the presence of the hymen may or may not always be proof of virginity.

107

First intercourse is always very painful and causes a lot of bleeding.

FACT:

The hymen's response to first intercourse depends upon its condition.

In some females, this tissue may be thin and almost nonexistent. Vigorous exercise may have disrupted it, such as cycling, horseback riding or inserting tampons. First intercourse therefore, may cause little or no pain and there may be slight to no bleeding. Some females however, have a thicker hymen. In these individuals disruption of the hymen may produce more pain or bleeding.

108

Premature ejaculation occurs only in young men.

FACT:

Premature ejaculation can occur at any age. It is a common form of sexual dysfunction in males. The timing of premature ejaculation is measured as the Intravaginal Ejaculatory Latency Time (IELT), from beginning of vaginal penetration until ejaculation. However, I had a patient whose ejaculation occurred as soon as he lowered his undershorts. Penetration was out of the question.

Some of the factors promoting premature ejaculation include:

- Early sexual experience
- Prostatitis
- Anxiety
- Fatigue
- Depression
- Neurological problems

Fortunately, premature ejaculation can usually be remedied.

109

Premature ejaculation means a man is having sex elsewhere.

FACT:

Premature ejaculation can occur whether or not sex is occurring elsewhere. If premature ejaculation occurs with one partner but not with another partner, then psychological factors are likely to be involved.

Other factors in premature ejaculation may include:

- Early sexual experience
- Prostatitis
- Anxiety
- Fatigue
- Depression
- Neurological problems

Most men have experienced premature ejaculation at some point in their lives. This can be a very frustrating experience for the man as well as his sexual partner.

A rare occurrence of premature ejaculation may not be significant. Recurrent or persistent premature ejaculation can be troubling, or in the least, embarrassing, and require the attention of an appropriate health care provider.

110

The rougher the man, the better the sex.

FACT:

I once heard a woman say that if she doesn't end up on the floor or under the bed, sex wasn't good enough.

Not every woman enjoys pain. Not every man likes the rough and tumble.

Some women have sadistic tendencies but most women like to be hugged, fondled, kissed, caressed and be handled as if she were something precious. Rough sex can result in unwanted injuries. Injury should not be a part of love making.

I have heard men boast of the discomfort caused during sex. Satisfaction was in the man's head, not in the woman's body. Some men think that gentle sex is no sex. Sometimes the condition of the female may require gentility.

111

A man would not enjoy sex with a woman who had a hysterectomy.

FACT:

Interestingly, most men cannot tell if a woman had a hysterectomy by having sex with her. There is nothing with a big H stamped on it. Sometimes it is difficult enough for a physician to tell if a woman has had this procedure let alone a man who is being intimate with her.

In most cases, sex with a woman after hysterectomy should be as enjoyable as before the hysterectomy. There are some cases where the surgery shortens the vagina, or scarring and chronic inflammation occur. These unusual situations can impact sexual activity.

Women have hysterectomies for sound medical reasons including cancer of the cervix and womb, fibroids (benign tumors), uterine prolapse and abnormal uterine bleeding. The operation may result in a total removal of the womb, which is called a total hysterectomy. Supracervical (or partial) hysterectomy involves removing the womb above the level of the cervix. Vaginally there is no difference compared to before the operation. A radical hysterectomy involves removal of the uterus and cervix as well as a portion of the upper vagina.

A man may have the odd notion that a woman who had a hysterectomy is not a complete woman. She is just as much a woman as he is a complete man. The surgery is done on her womb, not on her sexuality.

112

If a pregnant woman attempts to have sex with a man other than the baby's father, the baby wouldn't allow him to enter her. If the baby's daddy has sex with her, the baby would move aside and allow her to have sex.

FACT:

This is indeed an interesting myth. Interesting, but not true.

A developing fetus has no knowledge or control over worldly events. The neurologic system of the developing baby is not fully developed even at birth, let alone before birth. So, the baby is not aware of what the mother is attempting to do, let alone who she is doing it with.

Anatomically, the pregnant uterus is not involved in the sexual intercourse any way. Movement of the baby in the womb would not block anything going on in the mother's vagina.

113

The sex of a baby is determined by the position of the parents during sex.

FACT:

Ejaculated sperm and ovulated eggs have no concept of their contributor's position. Imagine a sperm travelling through a vagina, cervix, uterus, and through a fallopian tube where fertilization occurs, and that's after coming from a testicle, spending time in the epididymis, through a vas deferens, mixing in seminal fluid from the prostate gland and perhaps the seminal vesicle, then forcibly ejected through the urethra. That sperm couldn't care less about the sexual position of its originator. The chromosomes in the sex cells were determined before sex ever took place. Sexual positions have no relationship or influence in determining chromosomal makeup of an ovum or developing fetus.

In the case of artificial insemination there is no sexual position. This negates the idea of a baby's sex being determined by the sexual position of the parents. The sex of a baby is determined primarily by the chromosomal makeup in the sperm from the male. The female egg contributes an X chromosome. The sperm contributes an X or Y chromosome. An X from the egg combining with an X from the sperm will yield a female baby. An X from the egg combining with a Y from the sperm produce a male baby. Sexual positions have nothing to do with how the chromosomes combine.

114

Swallowing semen after oral sex is good because semen is very nutritious.

FACT:

Semen is nutritious for you, if you are a sperm!

Semen contains mostly fructose, enzymes, trace amounts of minerals and amines. These provide energy for the sperm and allow fertilization of the egg by the sperm. Semen is not a good source of proteins, as some believe. This is not recommended as a good addition to the adult human diet.

115

Spitting is safer than swallowing.

FACT:

This is suggestive of an attempt to avoid the transmission of disease. Sexually transmitted diseases can be contracted whether you spit or swallow.

The warm, moist environment of the mouth and throat is a good set up for the transmission of sexually transmitted diseases. Even only a short exposure of pathogens to mucosal membranes can result in the spread of disease.

Even if a person attempts to spit out infected material there may be pathogens left behind, or some may have already reached beyond the mouth before spitting takes place.

116

Penile warts are ticklers.

FACT:

This is a dangerous way to be tickled.

Penile warts, or condylomata, are caused by viruses. It is a viral infection and can be transmitted by sexual activity. These warts may be small or large, uncomfortable, or asymptomatic, unnoticeable, or obvious, external, or internal (in the urethra), even in the bladder and rectum.

The warts may seem innocuous but can cause problems. They can cause stinging, itching, burning, and bleeding if abraded. They can also cause obstruction of the urethra. If transmitted to females. they can obstruct the cervix which can result in infertility. In rare cases warts may undergo transformation and end up as a malignancy.

I saw a case where a young man's partner would not allow him to have "her ticklers" removed. She was playing with fire, perhaps unknowingly. Penile warts are not "French ticklers."

117

Frequent sex causes the vagina to stretch permanently.

FACT:

One of the characteristics of vaginal tissue is its resilience. After sex, and even after childbirth, the vagina resumes its normal configuration. The weakening of the pelvic muscles is known to occur due to multiple births and pelvic trauma. However, this is a different issue from vaginal integrity in normal sexual activities.

SEXUALLY TRANSMITTED DISEASES AND SEXUAL MYTHS

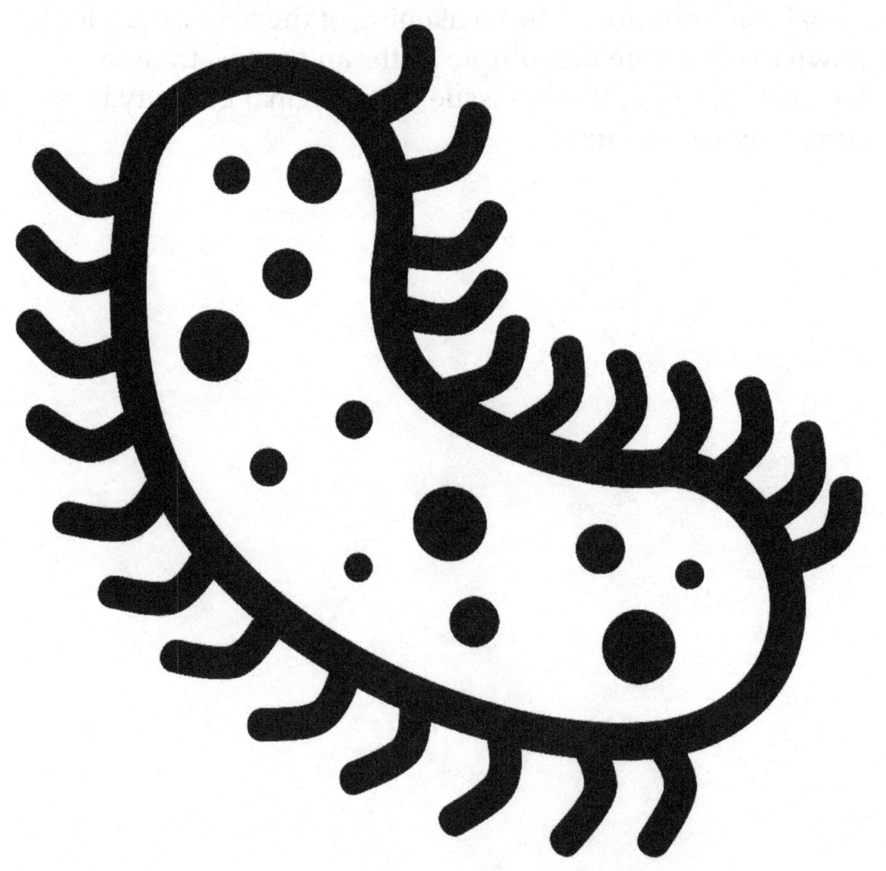

118

Safe sex prevents AIDS and other diseases.

FACT:

Many individuals consider using a condom as safe sex. There is no guarantee that a condom won't slip off or perforate during sexual activity. Safe sex must mean sex with a mutually healthy, faithful partner, or the safest of all, abstinence.

119

HIV/AIDS is a gay disease.

FACT:

Anyone can get AIDS. (Acquired Immunodeficiency Syndrome)

It was once thought that AIDS was a homosexual disease. It can be transmitted between gay people but also between heterosexual people as well. Any exchange of body fluids renders a person susceptible to contracting AIDS. Disease is no respecter of sexual orientation.

Transfusion of infected blood or blood products can also spread the disease.

120

Repeated exposure to HIV is required to get infected.

FACT:

One time is once too many.

Exposure to the pathogen risks entry into the body and this increases the dangers of contracting HIV. In a person, whose immune system is already compromised, it is even more likely that a single exposure can result in HIV infection.

Some "chances" are just not worth taking!

121

I won't get STD from someone I know.

FACT:

A sexually transmitted disease can be spread from anyone to anyone. Knowing a person has nothing to do with transmission of an infection.

122

Sex with a virgin cures venereal diseases.

FACT:

This is a vicious myth. It is sad enough to contract a venereal (sexually transmitted) disease. It is even more tragic to expose an innocent virgin to such devastation.

Having sex with a virgin does not treat or cure anything!

123

Having sex with a virgin will cure AIDS.

FACT:

This is one of the most ridiculous myths around.

AIDS is one of the most devastating of the sexually transmitted diseases. It requires intense medical attention and treatment. AIDS causes much misery, physically, medically, socially, and psychologically. The best cure is abstinence----not getting it in the first place.

Once AIDS is contracted, further sexual activity will only expose others to this dreaded disease. Sexual activity, especially with innocent virgins has nothing to do with curing AIDS, or anything else.

124

The contraceptive pill protects against STD's.

FACT:

The contraceptive pill (birth control pill) offers no protection against sexually transmitted diseases. The pill may be effective in preventing pregnancy but precautions must be taken to guard against exposure to these diseases. It is especially important for adolescents to understand that birth control pills have no antibiotic activity. They do not protect against any infection.

125

Herpes infection can only be transmitted by intercourse.

FACT:

Herpes infection can be transmitted by kissing and any other skin to skin contact.

126

Herpes can only be transmitted during an active outbreak.

FACT:

Herpes is the most contagious when an acute lesion is present, but it can also be spread when no active lesion is visible. It can be spread by touching, kissing, oral sex, anal sex, as well as by regular intercourse.

Herpes is especially dangerous during childbirth. If the baby's eyes become infected there may be catastrophic results. The immature neonate nervous system is also susceptible to the herpes virus.

127

A male is not mature until he has experienced the claps.

FACT:

As a youngster, I could never understand why some would think that having a disease would make a person "mature."

Experiencing sexually transmitted diseases is not a normal part of growing up. These diseases have acute and chronic effects in the body. The claps, also known as the whites, the drip, gentleman's disease, or gonorrhea, causes penile discharge, painful urination, bloody urination, prostatitis, pharyngitis from oral sex, arthritis, cardiac valvular disease, infertility, and many other ailments.

None of these ailments is required as a part of becoming a man. The claps has no role in a male's development physically, emotionally, or otherwise.

128

Oral sex is safe sex.

FACT:

There are individuals who think that any form of sexual activity other than vaginal penetration by the penis is safe sex. This is not true. Oral sex can be dangerous. It is no safer than any other form of sex. The mucosal lining of the oral cavity is susceptible to sexually transmitted diseases. These diseases can lead to a great morbidity and death rate. In fact, oral sex is implicated in the rise in oropharyngeal cancers (mouth and throat cancers) being seen in recent times.

There is evidence that the human papilloma virus (HPV) can cause oropharyngeal cancer. According to the U. S. National Cancer Institute there has been an increase in the incidence of HPV related oropharyngeal cancers, especially among males.

It is worth noting that tobacco and alcohol increase the risk of mouth and throat cancer when the human papilloma virus is present too.

If you have engaged in oral sex, consult a physician if you have any of the following:

- Persistent hoarseness or sore throat
- Persistent pain or difficulty swallowing
- A lump in the neck region
- Persistent sore in the mouth

The more sexual partners a person is involved with, the more likely there is for exposure to the human papilloma virus. So, the more oral sexual partners, the greater the chances of mouth and throat cancer.

129

Oral sex can prevent STD's.

FACT:

Don't bet on it!

The pathogens that cause STD's don't really care where they enter the body. Some bugs may have a propensity for certain parts of the body but the oral cavity is a welcoming port for many diseases.

Oral sex will prevent pregnancy, but it will do nothing to protect against sexually transmitted diseases. It will allow the transmission of Chlamydia, Gonorrhea, Herpes, Syphilis, Hepatitis B, Cytomegalovirus, HIV/AIDS, and many other diseases. I will never forget a case during my third year of medical school. An extremely beautiful woman presented with a hole in her palate (roof of the mouth). I was dismayed to learn her diagnosis-------Syphilis.

130

Promiscuity is always the cause of STD transmission.

FACT:

Not necessarily. Recent studies show that poverty and education are also important factors in the transmission of STDs.

Although promiscuity may not always be the cause of STD transmission it certainly plays a significant role in the spread of these diseases.

Consider the following: Mr. A is infected with disease X. He transmits the disease to Miss M on Saturday night. On Monday night Mr. A infects Mrs. Q. On Monday night Miss M infects Mr. P and Mr. T. Note that within two days disease X has been spread among at least four people. Sometimes a person can infect several people in a single night. Imagine the extent of damage that can occur in one month! This is the challenge of promiscuity.

Not all poverty-stricken people are promiscuous. Similarly, not all uneducated people are promiscuous. However, it is common knowledge that diseases like STD's tend to be more prevalent among the less fortunate and less informed individuals. Part of the reason for this may be the unfortunate quest for income among some poverty-stricken people.

Education is undoubtedly a key factor in combating this scourge. We all need to be well informed about the dangers of sexually transmitted diseases. Health Departments are generally doing a great job but much still remains to be done.

131

You can catch an STD from a toilet seat.

FACT:

Most unlikely. Most germs that cause STD's don't live for long periods outside of the body. They like warmth and moisture. Hard smooth surfaces, like a toilet seat, are hostile to these agents.

Good sanitation, though, is still the order of the day.

132

Sex in a swimming pool is safe because chlorine in the water will prevent STD's.

FACT:

Chlorine may be hostile to certain pathogens. However, ejaculation into the vagina can transmit STD's. Skin to skin contact allows transmission of diseases even in wet environments. Likewise, kissing in a pool is no guarantee of protection against oral transmission of disease.

133

You can only have one STD at a time.

FACT:

If you get an STD, you are more likely to have another. This is because the intimate environment that exposes a person to a sexually transmitted disease is likely to have more than one STD lurking around. Misery likes company!

For example, AIDS is not a single disease and that is why it is called a syndrome. It is a combination of diseases. This is one reason why it is so difficult to treat AIDS successfully using a single agent.

134

All STD's can be cleared up with antibiotics.

FACT:

STD's that are caused by bacteria can be treated with antibiotics. However, viral infections, e.g., herpes, & condylomata, cannot be successfully treated with antibiotics.

135

An STD will "burn out" eventually if left untreated.

FACT:

This is another very dangerous myth. An untreated sexually transmitted disease may have serious consequences for the infected individual. Some STD's may not have obvious symptoms, while some symptoms may seem to abate over time, even if the disease is not treated. This does not mean that the disease is gone or is no longer active in the body.

Some long-term effects of sexually transmitted diseases include the following:

- Social upheaval in homes
- Sterility in males and females
- Gonococcal arthritis
- Damaged heart valves
- Pelvic inflammatory disease in females
- Brain damage from syphilis
- HIV complications including death

MISCELLANEOUS SEXUAL MYTHS

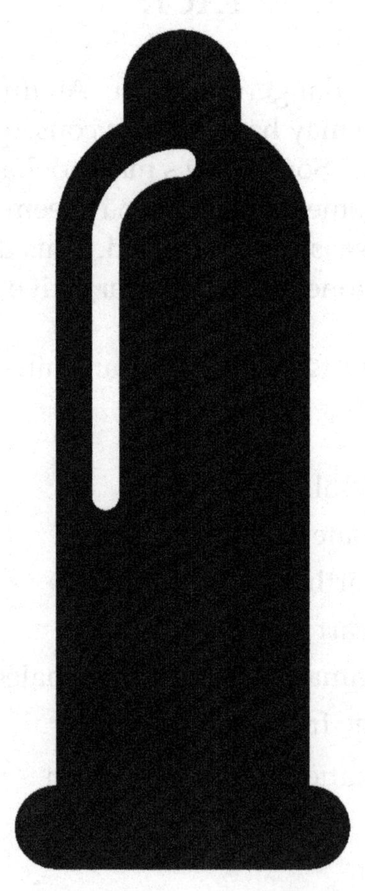

136

A homosexual can be easily identified.

FACT:

This myth is based on the belief that all homosexual males exhibit effeminate behavior. Outward appearance can hardly identify a person's sexual preference in most cases.

Persons with same sex preferences can be found amongst all professions, and walks of life. Age is no prohibitor either.

Today, there are many homosexual individuals who portray no given characteristics. Their chosen lifestyle is known only to themselves or specific individuals who they wish to share it with.

137

Only homosexuals have anal sex.

FACT:

Many heterosexuals engage in anal sex as well.

138

Sperm can by depleted by masturbation.

FACT:

Unlikely. Sperm are continuously produced, same as in a man
who has sex often. Note that nature has built-in recuperative
mechanisms, such as the refractory period in males. This is
the period of time, after ejaculation, during which ejaculation
will not occur again. It is evident that nature has ultimate
control in our bodies.

139

Vasectomy causes cancer.

FACT:

A vasectomy is the surgical interruption of the vas deferens,
the tubes that transport sperm from the testicles. This common
procedure is usually done to produce sterility in males. There
is no scientific evidence showing that a vasectomy is a
causative factor in the etiology of cancer.

140

Vasectomy causes impotence.

FACT:

Vasectomy results in sterility but not impotence. A man's potency should be the same after vasectomy as it was before the procedure. During vasectomy, the vas deferens are operated on. No other structures are involved in a vasectomy.

141

Foods change the taste of semen.

FACT:

Some claim that parsley, cinnamon, dairy products, cauliflower, broccoli, asparagus, alcohol and smoking can affect the taste of semen.

There is no scientific evidence that the food one eats determine the taste of semen. The taste of semen is more likely to be influenced by its contents whether that be alkalinity or acidity.

142

Taking birth control pills is a sign of promiscuity.

FACT:

Birth control pills are taken as a form of family planning, or, for the regulation of menstruation. Neither of these reasons have anything to do with promiscuity. A young woman taking birth control pills for family planning is showing signs of maturity.

A woman taking birth control pills for regulation of menses is generally a person concerned about her health and wellbeing. She is following the advice of her gynecologist or other health provider.

A promiscuous woman may have her own reasons for taking birth control pills, perhaps to avoid pregnancy. Not all women on birth control pills are promiscuous.

143

Eating a lot of okra during pregnancy produces an easy delivery.

FACT:

Okra has no bearing on the birth process. Nor will any other so called lubricant. No need to stock up on olive oil, K-Y jelly, WD-40 or otherwise.

144

Oral sex isn't really sex.

FACT:

Oral sex is an intimate activity just like vaginal sex. Many individuals think of it as being even more intimate than vaginal sex.

Oral sex involves undressing, close and intimate contact, and may lead to experimentation and creativity just as with other ways of having sex.

Along with the enjoyment of the activity there is also the risk of sexually transmitted diseases, such as Chlamydia, Gonorrhea, Herpes, Syphilis, Hepatitis B, Cytomegalovirus, HIV/AIDS, and many other diseases.

145

Getting pregnant for a blood relative causes the baby to be born mentally retarded or deformed.

FACT:

Not necessarily. A baby born to blood relatives may be quite normal. This happens every day. However, if an inheritable trait is passed onto the baby by both mother and father, it is more likely to see that trait manifest itself in the baby. There may be an increased chance of this occurring when pregnancy occurs between near relatives.

A congenital defect may occur due to genetics but not merely because the parents are related. If this were not the case, a lot of messed up kids would be seen in numerous elite families.

It should be noted that a mentally challenged or congenitally deformed child is not necessarily the product of sex between blood relatives and should not be viewed as such.
There is the potential for thousands of missteps during fetal development. A deficient mineral, amino acid or vitamin can affect the child's normal development. Here's an example: If the pregnant woman is deficient in folate, one of the B-complex vitamins, her child can be born with spinal problems.

146

Sex during pregnancy will cause miscarriage.

FACT:

Normal sex during pregnancy is usually safe and would not cause a miscarriage.

Up to 30% of pregnancies end in miscarriage.

There are many causes of miscarriage including the following:

- Lack of implantation of the embryo (developing baby) in the womb
- Abnormal development of the embryo (fetus)
- Chromosomal defects
- Autoimmune disorders. The mother's body may sense a problem in the developing baby. Her body may even recognize it as foreign to her own and dispel it (a miscarriage).

147

Over-reaching during pregnancy can cause the baby to be born with a broken neck.

FACT:

It is amazing that so many women believe this myth. Nothing can be further from the truth.

Stretching and over-reaching during pregnancy do not affect the fetal spinal cord. It is more likely to affect the spinal cord of the mother. The developing baby is well protected in the sac of fluid called the amnion and amniotic fluid. Injury to the baby is unlikely without trauma to the mother's abdomen. Manipulations during delivery of the baby are more likely to cause possible injury.

148

Wet dreams are a sexual disorder.

FACT:

Wet dreams, called nocturnal emissions, are normal occurrences.

A wet dream is a spontaneous orgasm during sleep. This may occur in males or females. In the male, ejaculation may occur. In the female, vaginal lubrication may occur. The exact trigger of wet dreams is not defined. It is not a sexual disorder or illness.

149

If a baby has plenty of head hair the mother would have heartburn.

FACT:

Heartburn is the symptom of chest or abdominal discomfort from the reflux of stomach acid into the esophagus. A baby's physical attributes have no bearing on the integrity of a mother's gastroesophageal sphincter, the mechanism that prevents the acid reflux.

It is difficult to find any logic in such a myth.

150

"Blue balls" is a life-threatening condition.

FACT:

When prolonged sexual stimulation without ejaculation occurs, a man may feel discomfort or pain in the testicular area. A light skinned male may see a bluish tint or discoloration through the skin of the scrotum.

Blue balls results from the congestion of prostatic and seminal fluids, vasocongestion of increased blood flow in the penis, and even the epididymis. When this congestion is prolonged without orgasm discomfort and pain can result. Fortunately, the pain resolves spontaneously and it is not a life-threatening matter.

151

Too much sex causes prostate cancer.

FACT:

Frequent sex does not cause prostate cancer.

The exact cause of prostate cancer, to date, has not been precisely delineated. Prostate cancer is a multifaceted problem. It is known that a high animal fat diet creates an increased risk for developing this disease.

It appears that animal fat serves as a reservoir for substances that may be implicated in causing prostate cancer. Abnormal fat metabolism is also suspected. Other risk factors for developing prostate cancer include age, race, demographics, hormonal levels and levels of minerals and vitamins.

Prostate cancer can occur in a man whether he is sexually active or not.

152

Cancer of the breast is caused by wearing tight bras.

FACT:

Many girls and adult females wear tight bras because they think it makes them appear sexy and more appealing to men. Tight bras, especially ill- fitting ones, may increase irritation of breast tissue. This is not likely to lead to breast cancer. More likely factors include a woman's genetic susceptibility, hormonal influences, diet, body vitamin and mineral deficiencies together with exposure to toxins, etc.

153

Marijuana stimulates strong erections.

FACT:

Marijuana may initially produce an increase in testosterone levels. This can allow a man to feel more macho, and have strong erections.

Unfortunately, marijuana can have the opposite effect after a while. I have seen men who were not only impotent from marijuana, but whose sperm count had also fallen to near zero.

Incidentally, upon cessation of marijuana use some sperm counts recovered but some did not. This suggests that marijuana may have long term and even permanent effects on the human body.

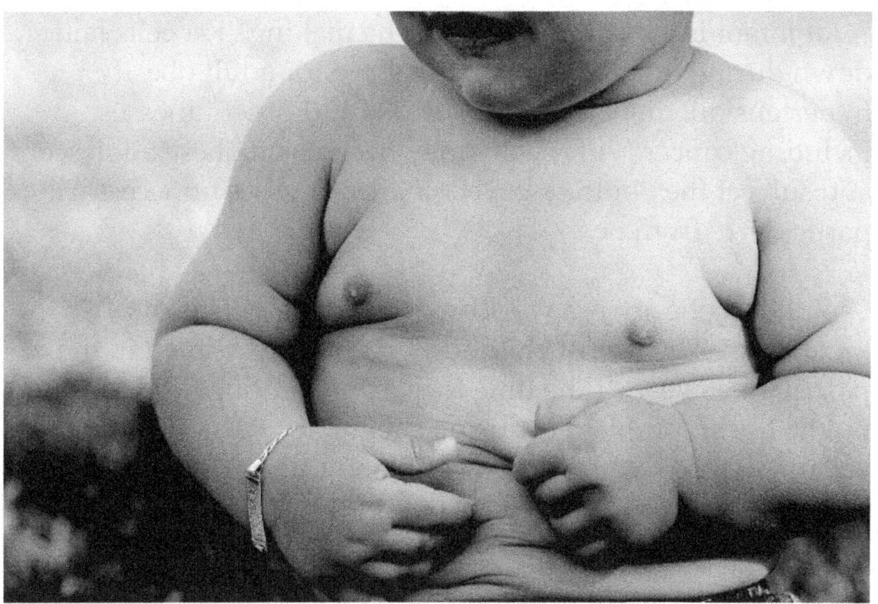

154

A fat baby is a healthy baby.

FACT:

This is a truly unfortunate myth.

A fat baby is more likely to be an unhealthy baby. Many people think that a jolly fat baby means that all is well with the child.

A fat infant is a health disaster in the making. Fat cells laid down during infancy may set the stage for adult obesity, hypertension, diabetes, heart disease and other illnesses, including cancer. A fat baby may become an obese adolescent and subject the youth to psychological stresses unnecessarily, particularly from peers.

Childhood obesity is a worldwide problem which is increasing. The rate of childhood obesity has tripled in the past 20 to 25 years. The time to start preventing this looming public health problem is during pregnancy (Watch what you eat and manage your weight well) and during the child's infancy.

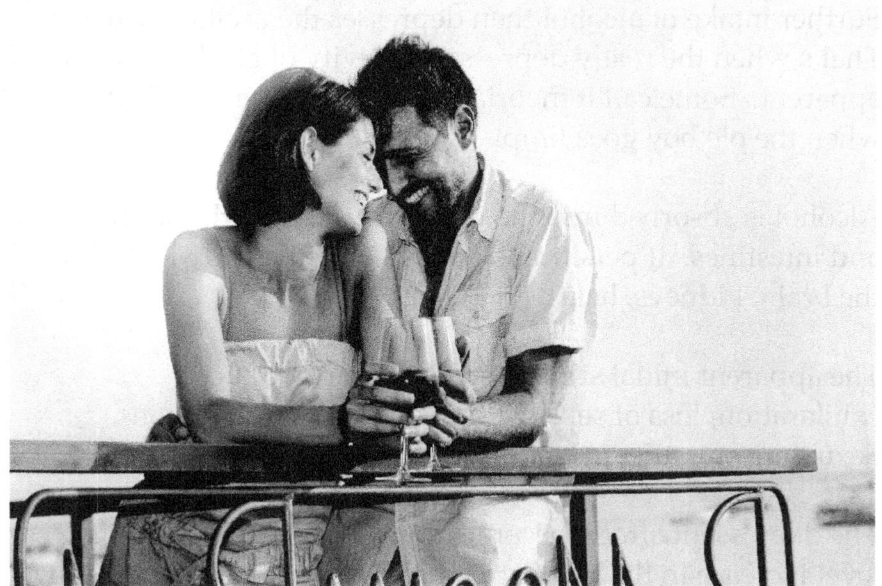

155

Alcohol is a sexual stimulant.

FACT:

This is a reference to "drinking" alcohol, also called ethanol. Alcohol is a depressant!

All nerves in the body either depress a function or increase (excite) a function. Initially, alcohol depresses nerves that depress activities, leaving excitatory nerves functioning. This gives the impression of a stimulant, whether sexual or otherwise.

Further intake of alcohol then depresses the excitatory nerves. That's when the really depressant activity of alcohol becomes apparent. Some call it inebriation or drunkenness. That is when the ole boy goes limp!

Alcohol is absorbed into the bloodstream from the stomach and intestines. It penetrates all organs of the body including the brain, kidneys, heart, and liver.

The apparent initial stimulant effects can produce exhilaration, loss of self-restraint and loss of inhibitions. Sexual promiscuity is common at this stage.

The depressant effects become more evident as the alcohol level increase in the bloodstream. This may manifest itself by loss of motor control (like stumbling on walking), loss of body functions, memory loss, blackouts and even death. Even if recovery occurs, there may be permanent injury to various organs of the body.

156

Alcohol makes sex better.

FACT:

This may or may not happen. Alcohol is a depressant.
However, a person's physical reaction to alcohol in any acute
situation may depend upon the individual. Eventually,
though, alcohol depresses bodily functions.
Alcohol can affect a man or woman's behavior during sex,
positively or negatively. It can also cause premature
ejaculation in some men.

157

Certain foods are aphrodisiacs.

FACT:

If this were true, the grocery stores would be busier than the movies.

There are no foods that universally get the sex juices flowing. I have heard some folk make claims for oysters, eggs, dark chocolates, sea urchins, conch, sardines, asparagus, almonds, bananas, ginger, guava, and many other food items.

Anything can turn a person on if he or she associates that item with sex.

158

Having sex reduces athletic performance.

FACT:

No truth to this. Some star athletes seem to be the horniest people around. Many high performing athletes got into trouble because of their sexual prowess.

If athletes allow sexual activities, or anything else, to interfere with their training routines and schedules, those activities may very well usurp performance. In such cases the problem is not the sexual activity, but, the lack of adherence to athletic guidelines, both mentally, and physically.

Many people think that the energy used during sex takes away from the available energy during athletic sports performance. The number of calories expended during sexual intercourse is miniscule compared to what is expended during most competitive sports. The physiology involved for competitive sports is different from what is used in sex.

The intense, repetitive and sustained muscular activities of competitive sports far outweigh those in male or female sexual activities. The trained mental astuteness in sports is not necessary for sex.

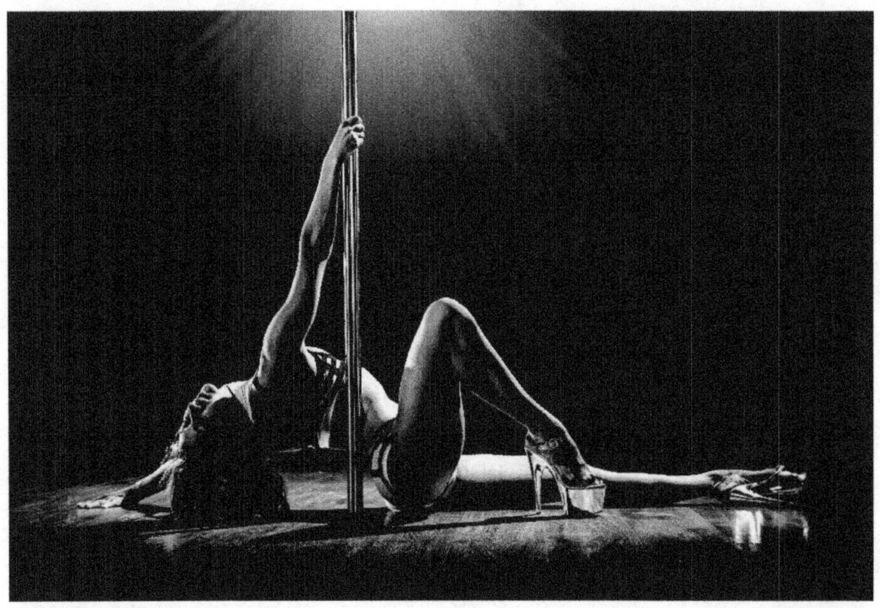

159

Good dancers make good sex partners.

FACT:

Not necessarily so. Being good on your feet doesn't automatically translate to being good between the sheets. Good sex is an achievement, and it does not happen every time intercourse takes place. Components of good sex include compatibility, desire, intimacy, communication, tolerance, and other such factors.

You cannot always dance around those components.

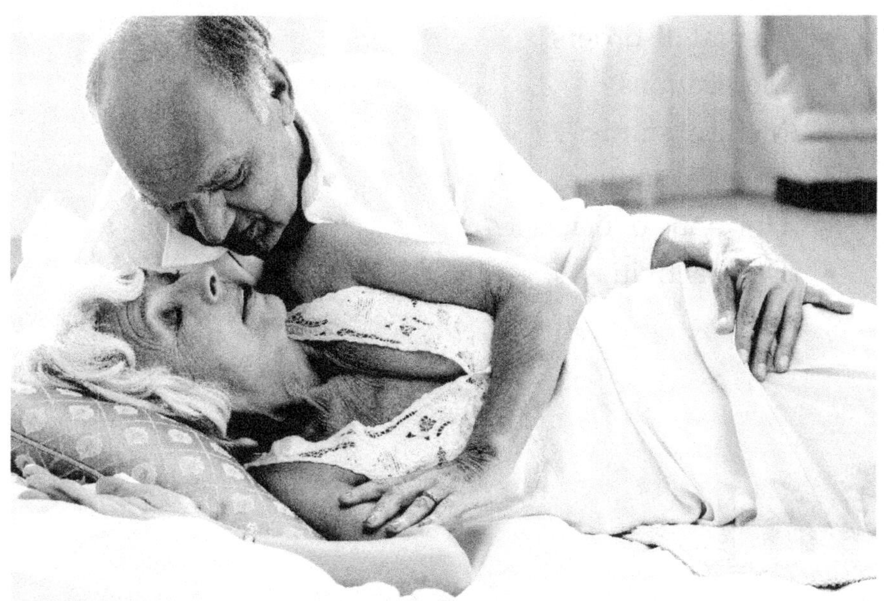

160

Losing interest in sex is a natural part of growing old.

FACT:

Not necessarily. Early in my urology practice, a 75 year old patient said to me, "I can do anything that you can do, maybe not as long as you can, but I can do it." His comment taught me a lesson.

Decreased libido in the elderly may be influenced by various factors including:

- Social conditions
- Separation of loved ones

- Mental disorders
- Medications
- Medical status
- Physical status
- Hormone deficiencies
- Daily activities

161

"If you never hit me you don't love me."

FACT:

It is amazing how many women actually believe this!
Some people confuse pain and pleasure. On the other hand,
some people appear to find pleasure in pain. It certainly
seems odd that inflicting pain could produce pleasure. I recall
observing a couple who lived nearby. They seemed to be the
ideal loving couple until exactly 5pm every Friday evening.
At exactly that time, they started fighting and fought
throughout the weekend until 8am Monday morning. The
wife often emerged on Mondays with bumps, bruises, and
swollen eyes.

Physical abuse is not necessary for expressing love, nor should
it be a component of sexual activity. It is amazing how many
women believe this myth, and, it is amazing how many men
try to oblige them.

Physical abuse is a poor way of expressing love. This can cause fear with erosion of love and romance. It also smacks of insecurity, jealousy, and lack of self- esteem. There is always the possibility of injury.

When I was in college there was a cute South American girl I was attracted to. One day she said to me, with tears in her eyes, "You don't love me because you've never hit me." That was the last conversation I had with her!

GLOSSARY

Abstinence: The total absence of sexual intercourse.

AIDS: Acquired immunodeficiency syndrome.

Amniotic fluid: The fluid in which the fetus (baby) develops in the womb.

Androgynous: The theory promulgated by Plato of the dual natures of male and female in primal creatures.

Andropause: The effects of declining androgen hormone levels in aging males.

Anorgasmia: The absence of orgasm during sexual intercourse.

Antibiotic: A medication used to fight infections.

Aphrodisiac: A favored substance that supposedly increases one's sexual desire.

Artificial insemination: The placement of sperm in the female reproductive tract without sexual intercourse.

Autoimmune disorder: A condition in which the body responds abnormally to native cells and tissues.

Azoospermia: The absence of sperm in semen or ejaculate.

Bacteria: A single celled organism that causes infections.

BCP: Birth control pills.

Birth canal: The passage from the cervix, through the vagina, through which a baby is born.

Blue balls: A painful condition involving inflammation of the epididymis.

Carrying angle: The characteristic angle at the elbow that usually distinguishes between male and female.

Cervix: The opening, or mouth, of the womb.

Chemotherapy: Any chemical used in the treatment of disease. This term is usually reserved for specific powerful mediations used in the treatment of serious illnesses.

Chromosome: The structures in sperm and eggs that contain genetic materials.

Circumcision: The surgical excision of redundant foreskin of the penis.

Clitoris: A usually sensitive structure above the urethral meatus in females.

Coitus: Sexual intercourse.

Coitus interruptus: The technique of withdrawing the penis from the vagina during sex, prior to ejaculation.

Conception: The time at which the sperm fertilizes the egg.

Condom: A sheath, usually latex, use to cover the penis to prevent pregnancy or disease.

Condyloma: A non-malignant growth thought to be caused by the condyloma virus.

Congenital defect: Usually refers to a malformation or dysfunction in the new-born.

Contraceptive: An agent used to prevent pregnancy.

Corpus cavernosa: Two of the three cylinders comprising the body (shaft) of the penis; the cylinders that contain spongy tissue that fill with blood during erections.

Corpus spongiosum: The third cylinder in the body of the penis that contains the urethra.

Cytomegalovirus: A common virus in the herpes group of viruses.

Dehydroepiandrosterone: Known as DHEA; a hormone produced in the adrenal glands; serves as a precursor of sex hormones in males and females.

Detumescence: Cessation of erection after ejaculation; can also happen abnormally during intercourse.

Diabetes mellitus: A body dysfunction in the handling of fat and sugar, characterized by low insulin production or the inability to properly utilize insulin.

DNA: Deoxyribonucleic acid, genetic material found in chromosomes.

Douching: Process of cleansing the vagina.

Dyspareunia: Painful sexual intercourse.

Egg: The sex cell that is produced by the ovary in females.

Ejaculation: The forceful ejection of semen from the penis during sexual intercourse.

Endocrine: The system of glands in the body that produce hormones.

Endometrium: The lining of the uterus or womb.

Episiotomy: An incision in the bottom of the vagina to accommodate childbirth.

Estrogen: The dominant hormone in females.

Fallopian tube: The passage through which the egg travels after release from the ovary, and the site of fertilization by the sperm.

Fertility: The ability to produce offspring.

Fertilization: The combination of sperm and egg that results in a developing fetus.

Fibroids: Non-malignant tumors of the uterus or womb.

Foreplay: Close interaction between a couple prior to sexual intercourse.

FSH: Follicle stimulating hormone.

Genetics: The science of inheritance.

Glans penis: The head of the penis, an expansion of the corpus spongiosum.

Gonococcal arthritis: Inflammatory changes in joints due to gonococcal infection.

Growth hormone: A hormone that regulates growth, produced by the pituitary gland in the brain.

Hemangioma: Considered to be a benign tumor, consisting of a cluster of abnormal blood vessels; often presenting as a birthmark.

Hematospermia: The presence of blood in the semen.

Hepatitis B: Inflammation of the liver caused by the Hepatitis B virus.

Herpes: A group of viruses in the Herpesviridae family.

HIV: Human Immunodeficiency Virus.

Hormone: A substance produced in the body that affects other parts of the body.

HPV: Human Papilloma Virus.

Hymen: A web of tissue at the vaginal introitus in sexually inactive females.

Hypertension: High blood pressure.

Hypogonadism: Deficient production of sex hormones.

Hysterectomy: The surgical removal of the uterus.

Impotence: The inability to achieve and maintain an erection that is satisfactory for sexual intercourse.

Infection: An abnormal effect of bacteria or viruses in the body.

Infertility: Incapable of producing or maintaining a pregnancy.

IUD: Intrauterine Device.

Libido: The interest or desire for sex.

LH: Luteinizing Hormone.

Mastectomy: The surgical removal of the breast.

Masturbation: Sexual self-stimulation.

Menopause: Changes in the aging female due to marked decrease in estrogen production.

Menorrhagia: Excessive bleeding during menstruation.

Menstruation: The bloody passage of the lining of the uterus, usually monthly, in the absence of pregnancy.

Metrorrhagia: Irregular bleeding from the womb.

Miscarriage: The spontaneous loss of pregnancy.

Mons pubis: A pad of fatty tissue over the bone that protects the urinary bladder.

Myth: A long standing incorrect belief.

Navel string: The umbilical cord.

Nocturnal emissions: Wet dreams; spontaneous orgasms during sleep.

Nuchal cords: Occurs when the umbilical cord is wrapped around the heck of the fetus.

Obstetrician: The physician who specializes in problems of the female reproductive system and the delivery of babies.

Oligospermia: A low sperm count.

Oophorectomy: The surgical removal of the ovaries and fallopian tubes.

Orgasm: The peak of sexual activity.

Ovary: Reproductive structure in females that produce eggs.

Ovulation: The release of eggs from the ovaries.

Oxytocin: An important hormone that is a active in the female reproductive system and milk production of in the breasts.

Pap smear: A diagnostic test on cells obtained from the cervix of the womb.

Pathogen: Any agent that produces a disease in humans.

Peyronie's disease: A placque found in the tunica layer of tissue in the penis.

Phenotype: Physical characteristics as inherited from parents.

Pornography: Explicit depiction of sex, sexual activities, and sexual paraphernalia.

Premature ejaculation: Release of semen sooner than desired.

Priapism: The prolonged, undesired penile erection.

Primal creatures: A nebulous form of ancient human existence, theorized by Plato and his followers.

Progesterone: A hormone produced by the ovaries, important in the menstrual cycle and pregnancy.

Prolactin: A hormone produced by the pituitary gland in the brain. It stimulates milk production in females and influences testosterone production in males.

Promiscuity: Sexual behavior that is generally unacceptable by society.

Prostate: The reproductive gland in the male pelvis that produces seminal fluid.

Prostate cancer: The malignant transformation of prostate cells.

Prostatitis: Inflammation of the prostate.

Rape: Forced, undesired and unwanted sexual activity.

Refractory period: The time after ejaculation during which a man cannot ejaculate again.

Retrograde ejaculation: The condition where semen is not ejected from the penis during orgasm, rather, falls back into the bladder. The semen is expelled during urination.

Semen: The combination of sperm from the testicles and seminal fluid from the prostate gland.

Semen analysis: A laboratory procedure for evaluating various parameters of semen.

Seminal fluid: The liquid portion of semen. produced by the prostate gland, contains nutrients for the sperm and serves as the transport medium for sperm.

Sexual dysfunction: Any abnormal sexual functioning in males or females.

Sperm: The sex cells produced by the testicles.

Sperm concentration: A measure of the number of sperm per cubic centimeter of semen.

STD's: Sexually transmitted diseases.

Stress: Medically, stress is physical, mental or emotional strain in response to a precipitating factor.

Symptom: Any complaint a person gives of a problem in the body.

Syphilis: A sexually transmitted disease caused by an organism called a spirochete.

Testosterone: The predominant hormone in males.

Tubal ligation: The interruption of the fallopian tube to prevent passage of the egg from the ovary.

Tunica albuginea: The tough layer of tissue surrounding the three anatomical cylinders in the penis and covering the testicles.

Umbilical cord: The tissue that connects the developing fetus to the placenta in the womb.

Undifferentiated stage of development: The developmental stage of the fetus when males and females physically appear to be similar.

Urethra: The channel through which urine passes from the bladder to the outside.

Uterus: The reproductive organ in the female.

Vagina: The physical space between the urinary bladder and the rectum. It serves as the sexual organ for intercourse and the birth canal for childbirth.

Vaginismus: The spontaneous contraction of vaginal tissues and pelvic muscles.

Vasectomy: The surgical interruption of the vas deferens.

Vasocongestion: The increased blood flow that results in swelling of tissues.

Venereal disease: A sexually transmitted disease.

Viagra: The original brand name for Sildenafil.

Virility: An expression of manliness.

Wet dream: A spontaneous orgasm occurring during sleep.

Made in the USA
Monee, IL
23 May 2024

58863126R00105